# Oncology
for Veterinary Technicians
and Nurses

# Oncology
## for Veterinary Technicians and Nurses

Editors

Antony S. Moore and Angela E. Frimberger

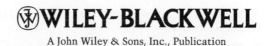

A John Wiley & Sons, Inc., Publication

Edition first published 2010
© 2010 Blackwell Publishing

Blackwell Publishing was acquired by John Wiley & Sons in February 2007. Blackwell's publishing program
has been merged with Wiley's global Scientific, Technical, and Medical business to form Wiley-Blackwell.

*Editorial Office*
2121 State Avenue, Ames, Iowa 50014-8300, USA

For details of our global editorial offices, for customer services, and for information about how
to apply for permission to reuse the copyright material in this book, please see our website at www.wiley.com/
wiley-blackwell.

*Library of Congress Cataloging-in-Publication Data*

Oncology for veterinary technicians and nurses / editors, Antony S. Moore and Angela E. Frimberger.
    p. ; cm.
  Includes bibliographical references and index.
  ISBN 978-0-8138-1276-2 (pbk. : alk. paper)
  1. Veterinary oncology.  2. Animal health technicians.  I. Moore, Antony S.  II. Frimberger, Angela E.
  [DNLM: 1. Neoplasms–veterinary.  2. Animals, Domestic.  3. Neoplasms–nursing.
4. Neoplasms–therapy.  SF 910.T8 O585 2010]
  SF910.T8.O53 2010
  636.089′6994–dc22

                    2009031845

A catalog record for this book is available from the U.S. Library of Congress.

Set in 10 on 12 pt Sabon by SNP Best-set Typesetter Ltd., Hong Kong
Printed in Singapore

1  2010

# Contents

# Acknowledgments

The people who have contributed the most to this book are the many veterinary technicians and nurses with whom we have both worked over our years in veterinary oncology. Many thanks are also due to our colleagues at the Animal Referral Hospital—and to the referring veterinarians who work with us through the Animal Referral Hospital and through our consulting service—for their ongoing support and productive conversations and for illustrations that many of them have contributed; thanks also to Jules Beatty for input on pain assessment. We thank the many wonderful clients and their beautiful brave pets that we have had the privilege of working with and who have taught us so much about medicine and more. Finally, we wish to thank those giving us permission to use illustrations in this book:

R. John Berg, DVM, Diplomate ACVS
Elizabeth Bertone-Johnson, ScD
Susan M. Cotter, DVM, Diplomate ACVIM (Oncology and Internal Medicine)
Anne G. Evans, DVM, Diplomate ACVD, MBA
Karl Kraus, DVM, Diplomate ACVS
Dennis J. Meyer, DVM, Diplomate ACVIM, Diplomate ACVP
Robert J. McCarthy, DVM, Diplomate ACVS
Nicole C. Northrup, DVM, Diplomate ACVIM (Oncology)
Gregory K. Ogilvie, DVM, Diplomate ACVIM (Oncology and Internal Medicine)
Dominique G. Penninck, DVM, DVSc, Diplomate ACVR and ECVDI
Kenneth M. Rassnick, DVM, Diplomate ACVIM (Oncology)
Pam Short, BVSc
David Simpson, BVSc, MVetClinStud, FACVS (Surgery)
Gordon H. Theilen, DVM, Diplomate ACVIM (Oncology and Internal Medicine)

# Contributors

Nicole Edwards, BSW
Social Worker
North Coast Cancer Institute
Port Macquarie, NSW, Australia

Lee Garrod, DACVECC
Diplomate of the American College of Veterinary Emergency and Critical Care Medicine
President of Veterinary Critical Care Veterinary Emergency, Critical Care and Cancer
  Treatment Center
Portsmouth, NH

Patricia Suomala B.S., CVT, M.Ed., CVPM
Director of Inpatient Services
MSPCA-Angell Animal Medical Center
Boston, MA

# Section Summary

**Section 1** discusses the process of cancer growth and spread and how cancer cells differ from normal cells; these chapters also give an overview of the causes of cancer, with epidemiologic information from the veterinary literature about cancers in cats and dogs.

**Section 2** presents pretreatment care of cancer patients. This includes biopsy and cytology to diagnose cancer, as well as the preferred technique to obtain information for a given patient, tissue handling, and submission guidelines to ensure that the best and most accurate results are obtained. These chapters also describe the testing needed to establish the extent of cancer in a patient (staging). This is of particular relevance to veterinary oncology nurses because they are often the ones performing the testing, and it underscores the importance of the results in making a prognosis and ensuring the best treatment choices for their patients.

**Section 3** broadly outlines the mainstream treatment strategies available in veterinary practice, including a brief discussion of alternative (complementary) treatments available.

**Section 4** is the most important for nurses because supportive care for patients is the area where nurses make a considerable difference to a pet dog or cat with cancer. Understanding supportive strategies for problems such as inappetence or pain is vital in the holistic treatment of the veterinary cancer patient.

**Section 5** discusses the support that can be so important to owners when they find their pet has been diagnosed with cancer. It also discusses the ethical concerns about treating animals with cancer as well as pet loss and the process of euthanasia. These chapters also discuss the important issue of the emotional impact of oncology practice for nurses.

**Section 6** describes the potential emergencies that can affect a patient with cancer, due either to their disease or to the treatment prescribed. It also outlines the interventions needed in these patients so that a nurse can be prepared before seeing the pet. This section is structured in a quick-reference format, with plenty of bullet lists and tables.

**Section 7** considers some of the most common cancers, in the form of case-based examples, that the veterinary nurse is likely to encounter. Included are summary information about the disease and prognostic factors, as well as the treatment of choice, adjunctive strategies to consider, supportive care needed, and palliative options.

**Section 8** contains reference points for nurses in the form of quick-reference charts of important information that nurses can access in a hurry.

...this book also offers assistance in more friendly, perhaps a good to start to a great partnership: the veterinary cancer patient.

If you are reading this book, you already understand that cancer is a common — too common — disease in our pets. You may — or may not — also know that cancer treatment most often results is less toxic and more compatible with a good quality of life than it is in some human patients. It also requires you, as a veterinary technician, to become more involved in the humane-animal bond than any other subspecialty of veterinary medicine. When working with cancer patients, you are truly a nurse, and not a technician. In fact you will notice that in this book we use the terms interchangeably, and encourage you to embrace the importance of nursing in our veterinary cancer patients.

Working as part of a veterinary cancer treatment team brings immense rewards. It soon becomes obvious that cancer is "the most treatable" of all chronic diseases, and that you, as a trained veterinary nurse provide services that are an integral part of an interdisciplinary approach to cancer care. You will find that although many of your patients are "terminal," you can provide continuous comfort to them, and their owners/caregivers, and that you will build relationships with both that are deep and often long lasting. You will cry when many of your patients die, but they will not be tears of frustration or anger. They will be tears shed from truly missing a patient and friend.

We hope that from the initial chapter to the end of the book we can help you achieve and promote excellence in cancer care through your professional contribution as a veterinary cancer nurse.

Antony S. Moore
Angela E. Frimberger

# Introduction

Although intended primarily for the nurse/technician who is working in a specialty practice, this book also offers technicians in general/family pet practice a guide to the integrated practice of nursing the veterinary cancer patient.

If you are reading this book, you already understand that cancer is a common and often deadly disease in our pets. You may—or may not—also know that cancer treatment in animals is less toxic and more compatible with a good quality of life than it is in some human patients. It also requires you, as a veterinary technician, to become more involved in the human-animal bond than any other subspecialty of veterinary medicine. When working with cancer patients, you are truly a nurse, and not a technician. In fact you will notice that in this book, we use the terms interchangeably and encourage you to embrace the importance of nursing in our veterinary cancer patients.

Working as part of a veterinary cancer treatment team brings immense rewards. It soon becomes obvious that cancer is "the most treatable" of all chronic diseases, and that you, as a focused veterinary nurse provide services that are an integral part of an interdisciplinary approach to cancer care. You will find that although many of your patients are "terminal" you can provide enormous comfort to them and their owners/caregivers, and that you will build relationships with both that are deep and often long-lasting. You will cry when many of your patients die, but they will not be tears of frustration or anger. They will be tears shed from truly missing a patient and friend.

We hope that from the initial chapter to the end of the book we can help you achieve and promote excellence in cancer care through your professional contributions as a veterinary cancer nurse.

Antony S. Moore
Angela E. Frimberger

# Oncology
## for Veterinary Technicians
## and Nurses

# Section 1

Basics of Oncology

# Introduction to Clinical Veterinary Oncology

## What Is Cancer?

Cancer is the process where normal cells in the body become transformed to undergo excessive or unrestrained growth. Cancer can occur in any bodily organ and can travel from one part of the body to another distant part by the blood or lymph system. There are more than 100 different types of cancer that can be grouped into one of several major categories.

**Sarcomas** are cancers that begin in tissue that connects, supports, or surrounds other tissues and organs (such as muscle, bone, and fibrous tissue). Examples include fibrosarcoma (malignant tumor of fibrocytes), hemangiosarcoma (malignant tumor of blood vessels), and osteosarcoma (malignant tumor of bone).

**Carcinomas** are cancers that originate in tissues that cover a body surface, line a body cavity or make up an organ. Carcinomas that derive from glandular tissue are prefixed with *adeno*. Examples include mammary adenocarcinoma (tumor of mammary glands) and transitional cell carcinoma (malignant tumor of bladder or urethra lining).

**Sarcomas and carcinomas** together are sometimes referred to as *solid tumors*.

**Lymphomas** are cancers that occur in cells that make up an important component of the immune system and protect the body's cells. Lymphomas are characterized by the *type of lymphocytes* forming the cancer (B-cell or T-cell) and by the *grade of the lymphoma* (low-grade vs. intermediate- to high-grade lymphoma).

**Leukemias** are cancers that occur in the blood-forming tissues and blood cells. Leukemias can be *acute* (high-grade and rapidly progressive), or *chronic* (low-grade and often slow to progress if treated).

**Leukemias and lymphomas** both belong to the "hematopoietic tumors" or "hematopoietic neoplasias."

5

## Communicating with Owners of Pets with Cancer

Veterinary clients often find veterinary technicians and nurses more approachable and easier to communicate with than the veterinarian, and you will find clients asking you questions that you may not be sure how to handle. First, it is important to clarify, with the veterinarian with whom you are working, how much direct communication you should undertake and whether there are any topics or advice that you should specifically seek to cover or avoid. Some veterinarians are happy to have technicians and nurses take on as much client communications as possible, whereas others prefer to handle communications themselves. It is important to keep this key working relationship harmonious, so be sure that you are in agreement with the person you are working with as to who will handle which part of communications.

Veterinary technicians and nurses are often in a position to discuss the fears and doubts that an owner has, even before cancer is diagnosed and characterized (usually by biopsy). Try as they might, when pet owners hear the word "malignant," it's hard to focus on anything but what it may mean for their pet. Common questions are: What are the treatment options? What will work? How will having cancer affect my pet's quality of life?

First, it is important to explain that the answers to most of these questions hinge on the specific diagnosis. Most cancers require more than one form of treatment to effectively fight the disease. This can mean using as many as four different cancer therapies, including surgery (surgical oncology), chemotherapy (medical oncology), radiation therapy (radiation oncology), and biologic response modifiers including immunotherapy. This requires a multidisciplined cancer care team that develops, coordinates, and monitors all aspects of an individual pet's treatment plan. You, as a veterinary technician (or more realistically in this setting, nurse) are critical to the successful functioning of this team.

**Suggest that owners collate their pet's medical history.** Particularly if owners are seeing a specialist veterinarian for the first time, it's important for them to give a complete picture of the health status of their pet. If the pet has several health problems or a long history with one, it can help the owner if you collate a history of events, recurrences, treatments, medications, and outcomes associated with the condition that you have on file; then suggest that the owner add to that record with his or her own recollections of the pet's medical history. If you are working in a referral hospital, collect as much data as possible from the owner, including the contact information from any veterinarian that may have information on file. A written list can save time and ensure completeness.

**Make sure all members of the cancer care team are informed.** If a patient develops a condition that requires one or more specialists or needs surgery, it's important that all members of that pet's veterinary medical team have complete and consistent information. Encourage owners to share the names and contact numbers of any others involved with the pet's care and bring all records with them.

**Tell the owners when and how they will receive test results.** Often owners are confused and impatient after tests have been ordered. Giving owners realistic timelines for them to be notified of test results and letting them know how they will receive them will allay a lot of this concern. Remember to tell them that if results do not arrive when they expect them, they should contact their veterinarian and inquire. A dedicated oncology technician may take on the role of contacting owners when test results are in and scheduling time for them to discuss the results with their veterinarian.

A common question from owners is "how is my pet likely to respond to treatment for cancer?" For cancer in dogs and cats, expected remission times and life span, or *prognosis*, is highly variable and depends on a number of factors, the most important of which is the *type* of cancer as diagnosed by biopsy. Untreated pets with malignant cancer often live 2 months or less, but this varies greatly depending on the type of tumor. With therapy, most dogs with lymphoma or osteosarcoma (two common cancers in dogs) will live 9 months to 1 year. Therefore, a reasonable goal is a 1-year survival. Occasionally the pet will live much longer, up to 2.5 years or more, and some will live out their normal lifespan. Some animals are truly cured of cancer, but this depends greatly on the tumor type. Other factors that will influence an individual pet's prognosis include

1. The stage (or extent) of the disease, which reflects the number, location, and size of major populations of tumor cells in the body.
2. Whether the pet is feeling sick or not. In general, pets that are not feeling sick and are diagnosed early in the course of tumor growth have a better chance of remission with treatment. Loss of appetite is an important symptom for all cancers, particularly if accompanied by unplanned, significant (>15%) weight loss.
3. Histologic grading: the specific appearance of tumor cells and their pattern of infiltration in various tissues (what the pathologists reports from a biopsy specimen).
4. The presence of paraneoplastic syndromes (tumor-associated conditions), such as high blood calcium (hypercalcemia).
5. The treatment chosen and the care given by the owner and veterinary cancer treatment team.
6. The pet's response to therapy. It is never possible to accurately predict the future for a given individual pet. Although it may be possible to predict the likelihood of achieving remission or long-term survival, ultimately the only remission that will matter to pet owners will be their own pet's—whether it fits in with the expected statistics or not. In many situations the only way to know whether a particular patient will benefit from treatment is to make an attempt.

## Specialist Veterinary Care

Although a primary care veterinarian is an integral part of the cancer care for any pet, pets with cancer may need to visit an expert in a specific area of veterinary medicine. These veterinarians have undertaken further training and have achieved certification by various veterinary Colleges. They are often called *specialists*.

Medical oncology is the general study and treatment of cancer. Medical oncologists are trained in the prevention, detection, and medical treatment of all forms of cancer. In the U.S. such specialists are certified by the American College of Veterinary Internal Medicine (ACVIM) subspecialty of Oncology: in Europe, by the European College of Veterinary Internal Medicine (ECVIM) subspecialty of Oncology; and in Australia by the Australian College of Veterinary Scientists (ACVSc).

Surgical oncology is the specialty concerned with the physical removal of cancerous tissue. Sometimes, surgery is augmented with other forms of care, such as chemotherapy or radiation therapy. Surgical oncologists have specialty experience in treating distinct types of cancer—from breast, bone, and lung cancer to cancers that occur within the abdomen, as well as skin cancer. Surgical specialists in the U.S. are certified by the American College of Veterinary Surgery (ACVS). Some of these specialists continue with Fellowships specifically in surgical oncology; there is no formal qualification for such specially trained individuals, but they are obviously the most highly trained surgeons performing cancer surgery.

Radiation oncology is the specialty concerned with prescribing radiation therapy in all its forms. In the U.S., radiation oncologists are certified by the American College of Veterinary Radiology (ACVR), subspecialty of Radiation Oncology.

Internal medicine deals with the function of the internal organs, such as the liver, kidney, and lungs, plus the diagnosis and treatment of associated problems. Internists often provide the first contact for an unspecified internal illness or problem. They may diagnose and treat the problem themselves or work in conjunction with another specialist (such as a medical oncologist) for more focused diagnosis and treatment. In the U.S. such specialists are certified by the American College of Veterinary Internal Medicine (ACVIM).

Emergency and critical care medicine is the specialty that deals with critical health and accident cases, where immediate treatment can sometimes mean the difference between life and death. In the U.S., such specialists are certified by the American College of Veterinary Emergency and Critical Care (ACVECC).

Veterinary technicians and nurses can achieve specialty qualifications also. The Academy of Internal Medicine for Veterinary Technicians promotes interest and advanced skills in the discipline of internal medicine. It is possible to become credentialed and recognized in the discipline of Veterinary Oncology. Candidates fulfill 3 years of experience, continuing education, and complete an examination. This qualification is available in the U.S.A., but it is possible for candidates from other countries to apply and qualify. http://aimvt.com/

# Causes of Cancer in Pets

## Epidemiology and Cancer

One of the most common questions clients ask is, "What caused my dog or cat's cancer?" That question is difficult to answer, but as in humans, the etiopathogenesis (cause and progression) of cancer in animals often involves both genetic and environmental risk factors. Indeed, some dog and cat breeds (Bernese mountain dogs, Siamese cats) have a high rate of cancer when compared to other breeds and are often susceptible to very specific kinds of cancers. In addition, exposure to cigarette smoke, asbestos, and other environmental contaminants has been associated with an increased risk of developing cancer in pets. Therefore, the prevention of cancer is based on the identification of animals that are at risk based on familial/genetic and environmental influences. Epidemiology is the science that examines these genetic and environmental influences that can then be used to reduce cancer risk.

The identification of factors associated with an increased risk of developing cancer is in its infancy in veterinary epidemiology and oncology. Despite this early state of development, several important observations have been made and are summarized in the following section. Clients should be educated that increased risk may not be equated with causality. In other words, exposure to a risk factor may not have *caused* their pet's cancer; however; such studies can still act as a guide for the concerned owner.

## Causes of Cancer in Pets

### Nutrition

A lifetime study of restricted daily intake of the same food was done with a total of 48 Labrador retriever dogs from seven litters that were divided into two groups: one group

9

fed normally (control) and one group fed 25% less (restricted). The median life span of the restricted group was significantly longer. Although the overall prevalence of cancer between groups was similar, the mean age due to cancer-related deaths was 2 years later in the dogs that received the restricted diet. In another study, increased consumption of green leafy vegetables and yellow-orange vegetables (squash, carrots) decreased the risk of urinary bladder transitional cell carcinoma in genetically predisposed dogs.

Some practical suggestions for concerned dog owners might be to restrict daily intake from early maturity to allow their pet to maintain a thin body weight throughout life. Although it may not apply to all dogs and all cancers, it may be prudent to supplement their diet with leafy green or yellow-orange vegetables at least 3 times per week (as in the above study of bladder cancer in Scottish terriers).

Cats fed canned food have an increased risk of developing oral squamous cell carcinoma (SCC). Also, cats that eat more than 50% of their diet as canned cat food have an increased risk of developing a thyroid adenoma. Supplementation of diet with beef or poultry seemed to decrease the risk of hyperthyroidism in one study and could be suggested to concerned owners of cats.

## Spaying and Neutering

Spaying (ovariohysterectomy) has long been demonstrated to be a markedly effective method of preventing mammary tumors if it is performed before the first estrus. Spaying is moderately effective if performed before the dog is 2.5 years of age. Castration (orchiectomy) reduces the risk of testicular tumors, but not prostate cancer.

However, the effect of spaying and neutering (gonadectomy) may not always be protective. A study of Rottweiler dogs was conducted to study the effect of elective gonadectomy and the spontaneous development of appendicular bone sarcomas. In that study male and female Rottweiler dogs that underwent gonadectomy before 1 year of age were significantly more likely to develop bone sarcoma than dogs that were sexually intact.

## Genetics

A number of clear breed predilections have been demonstrated in veterinary oncology. German shepherd dogs have been shown to have bilateral cystadenocarcinomas and cutaneous fibrosarcomas. Flat-coated retrievers and Bernese mountain dogs have been shown to have a high incidence of cancer, especially malignant histiocytosis. Scottish terriers, especially those with exposure to herbicides have an increased risk of developing transitional cell carcinomas of the bladder. Siamese cats are prone to develop mammary carcinomas, intestinal carcinomas, and mast cell tumors of the skin; in contrast they are at low risk of developing thyroid adenomas and squamous cell carcinomas of the skin.

## Environmental Carcinogens

In sharing their living environment with humans, pets are exposed to many of the same environmental contaminants as their owners, including passive environmental tobacco smoke (ETS) ("second-hand smoke"). In fact, exposure levels in animals kept indoors continuously may be higher than those of human household members, who often spend extended periods of time outside the home. Metabolites of nicotine have been found in the urine of cats living with smokers and are higher than levels in humans exposed to ETS (Figure 2.1). Routes of ETS exposure in cats and dogs may be through inhalation and oral ingestion of contaminants deposited on the fur during grooming.

Dogs have been shown to have an increased risk of developing cancer of the respiratory tract, especially of the lung and nasal cavity when exposed to coal and kerosene heaters and ETS. One veterinary study found a weak association between lung cancer and exposure to tobacco in the home (odds ratio 1.6), but no dose-response relationship. The risk for developing lung cancer rose for dogs with short or medium-length nasal cavities. In a similar study, dogs of long-nosed breeds had an increased risk of developing nasal cancer when exposed to ETS than did dogs of breeds with shorter noses.

Cats exposed to ETS have a higher risk of developing lymphoma. Because domestic cats groom extensively, their alimentary tract, particularly the oral cavity, may be exposed to toxins deposited on their fur. These may include chemicals present in applied products such as flea powders and those present in environmental contaminants such as cigarette smoke. The most common site for oral SCC in cats is the ventral aspect of the tongue caudal to the lingual frenulum. Because of anatomy, this site is likely to accumulate irritant chemicals and carcinogens. Cats wearing flea-control collars have a higher risk of developing oral SCC, and those living with a smoker have a mildly increased risk.

Mesothelioma is more common in dogs owned by people who worked in the asbestos industry.

Lymphoma was more common in dogs that lived in an urban environment in one study. In addition, the use of chemicals by owners, specifically the commonly used lawn care herbicide 2,4-D, paints, asbestos or solvents, as well as radiation and electromagnetic field exposure have been associated with increased risk for canine lymphoma.

Application of insecticides (but not in a spot-on formulation) increased the risk of bladder cancer in Scottish terriers in another study.

It is impossible to be able to prevent cancer in all of our pets, but some options you can suggest to the concerned owner would be to reduce exposure to environmental carcinogens such as pesticides, coal, or kerosene heaters, and avoid the excessive use of lawn herbicides such as 2,4-D. For owners who are smokers, they should know there is a risk to their pets from environmental tobacco smoke. If possible, exposure to radiation and strong electromagnetic fields should be minimized. These steps may be particularly important for owners of susceptible breeds (for example a Scottish terrier with fleas should be treated with

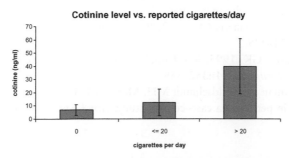

**Figure 2.1.** Urine cotinine (a metabolite of nicotine) was measured in urine of cats that did not live with a smoker, lived with a smoker that smoked fewer than 20 cigarettes a day, and lived with a smoker that smoked more than 20 cigarettes a day. The cotinine levels rose with level of exposure, and in the highest exposure group, cotinine levels approached those of *active* human smokers. (Courtesy of Dr. Elizabeth Bertone)

spot-on insecticides, rather than dips or sprays, which are shown to increase the risk of this cancer).

## Summary

Often a patient with cancer has none of the risk factors listed above. For owners of these pets, it may still be comforting to know what the risk factors are, and that their other pets will not be exposed to any of them. It may also provide an incentive to reduce exposure to known risk factors such as insecticides or ETS.

## Further Reading

Bertone ER, Snyder LA, Moore AS. 2002. Environmental tobacco smoke and risk of malignant lymphoma in pet cats. *Am J Epidemiol* 156:268–273.

Bukowski JA, Wartenberg D, Goldschmidt M. 1998. Environmental causes for sinonasal cancers in pet dogs, and their usefulness as sentinels of indoor cancer risk. *J Toxicol Environ Health A* 54(7):579–591.

Cooley DM, Beranek BC, Schlittler DL, et al. 2002. Endogenous gonadal hormone exposure and bone sarcoma risk. *Cancer Epidemiol Biomarkers Prev* 11(11):1434–1440.

Gavazza A, Presciuttini S, Barale R, et al. 2001. Association between canine malignant lymphoma, living in industrial areas, and use of chemicals by dog owners. *J Vet Intern Med* 15(3):190–195.

Glickman LT, Domanski LM, Maguire TG, et al. 1983. Mesothelioma in pet dogs associated with exposure of their owners to asbestos. *Environ Res* 32(2):305–313.

Glickman LT, Raghavan M, Knapp DW, et al. 2004. Herbicide exposure and the risk of transitional cell carcinoma of the urinary bladder in Scottish terriers. *JAVMA* 224(8):1290–1297.

Hayes HM, Tarone RE, Cantor KP. 1995. On the association between canine malignant lymphoma and opportunity for exposure to 2,4-dichlorophenoxyacetic acid. *Environ Res* 70(2):119–125.

Lawler DF, Evans RH, Larson BT, et al. 2005. Influence of lifetime food restriction on causes, time and predictors of mortality of dogs. *JAVMA* 226:225–231.

Raghavan M, Knapp DW, Dawson MH, et al. 2004. Topical flea and tick pesticides and the risk of transitional cell carcinoma of the urinary bladder in Scottish terriers. *JAVMA* 225:389–394.

Reif JS, Bruns C, Lower KS. 1998. Cancer of the nasal cavity and paranasal sinuses and exposure to environmental tobacco smoke in pet dogs. *Am J Epidemiol* 147(5):488–492.

Reif JS, Dunn K, Ogilvie GK, Harris CK. 1992. Passive smoking and canine lung cancer risk. *Am J Epidemiol* 135(3):234–239.

Reif JS, Lower KS, Ogilvie GK. 1995. Residential exposure to magnetic fields and risk of canine lymphoma. *Am J Epidemiol* 141(4):352–359.

Sonnenschein EG, Glickman LT, Goldschmidt MH, McKee LJ. 1991. Body conformation, diet, and risk of breast cancer in pet dogs: a case–control study. *Am J Epidemiol* 133(7):694–703.

# Section 2

## Approaching the Cancer Patient

# Diagnosis of Cancer

**3**

Being able to obtain diagnostic samples and establish definitive diagnoses is crucial to developing an effective treatment plan for a pet with cancer. Although veterinary oncology technician-nurses may not be directly involved in making a diagnosis, they are often called upon to handle and submit specimens from patients with cancer. Knowing how to correctly prepare these samples can be crucial in obtaining a reliable diagnosis, and in making a treatment plan for the patient.

As discussed previously, it is impossible to formulate a rational prognosis and treatment plan for a patient without knowing the definitive diagnosis of tumor type. This can not be done visually or by palpation and absolutely requires pathology testing.

The two main areas of pathology important in cancer diagnostics are *cytopathology* and *histopathology*. Cytopathologists are specialists at examining individual cells obtained by fine-needle aspirate or impression smear to determine the identity of a disease process. Histopathologists examine intact tissue samples and associated architecture to determine the underlying pathologic process. Choosing either diagnostic modality, or both, to apply in a given pet with cancer depends on the individual case variables. Some of the advantages and disadvantages of cytopathology compared to histopathology are summarized in Table 3.1.

The evaluation of cytological and histological samples both require specialized training and experience to obtain reliable results. Accuracy may be further improved upon or corroborated by more specialized techniques such as electron microscopy, polymerase chain reaction (PCR) and flow cytometry, which are becoming more widely available and will become an important part of veterinary diagnostics depending on the clinical situation. The type of sample required to perform these tests and test availability varies, and your pathology laboratory will be able to advise you if you are asked to submit samples from your patient.

The veterinary cancer nurse should be able to complete the submission form, including all relevant clinical information that will ensure that the pathologist has the best chance of making an accurate diagnosis. Most nurses should have a good understanding of the basic terms used in a pathology report (Table 3.2).

15

**Table 3.1.** Summary of the relative advantages of cytology and histopathology as diagnostic aids for pets with cancer

| Cytology | Histopathology |
|---|---|
| Can be used to screen patients for more comprehensive diagnostic tests. | Generally more accurate and more representative of the tissue of concern than fine-needle aspiration cytology. |
| Sample collection can easily be done preoperatively, often in the examination room without general anaesthesia or even without sedation, and is less likely to result in adverse effects when compared to tissue biopsy. | Provides information on tissue architecture that cannot be obtained from cytological specimens. In some neoplasms evaluation of tissue architecture/tissue invasion is essential to differentiate between benign and malignant neoplasms (e.g., mammary tumors). |
| Less costly than surgical biopsy in both sample collection and laboratory analysis. | The relatively large tissue sample provided by biopsy enables further specialized testing such as histochemistry (special stains), immunohistochemistry, electron microscopy, and polymerase chain reaction to be performed, if required, to achieve a definitive diagnosis. |
| Requires less sample processing than histopathology and thus provides earlier results than histopathology. | Histopathology is generally more likely to provide a definitive diagnosis, although the "investment" in time, client cost, and invasiveness of sample collection is greater. |

**Table 3.2.** Common terms found in pathology reports and their definition

| | |
|---|---|
| Tumor | Mass or swelling that may or may not be neoplastic; however, in normal use it generally refers to a neoplasm. |
| Hyperplasia | Increase in the number of cells present. |
| Metaplasia | Abnormal transformation of a differentiated tissue of one tissue type into differentiated tissue of another type. |
| Dysplasia | Abnormal change in the microscopic characteristics of a tissue that may be a preneoplastic condition. |
| Neoplasia/neoplasm | Abnormal benign or malignant growth that is not responsive to normal growth control. |
| In situ | Malignancy that is restricted to the superficial tissue and has not yet invaded below the basement membrane into underlying tissue. |
| Adenoma/papilloma | Benign neoplasm of epithelial origin. |
| Carcinoma | Malignant neoplasm of epithelial origin. |
| Adenocarcinoma | Malignant neoplasm of epithelial origin that is forming gland and ducts. |
| Sarcoma | Malignant neoplasm of mesenchymal origin. |
| Pleomorphism | Presence of multiple shapes and forms of cells and nuclei. |
| Anaplasia | Total loss of microscopic characteristics of differentiation. |
| Scirrhous response | Abundant fibroblastic proliferation with collagen formation in response to invasive malignant tumors. |

# Tumor Cytology

Cytology is relatively simple to perform, and sample collection is minimally invasive for peripheral sites. For these reasons it can be a useful screening tool, avoiding surgical biopsy of benign (e.g., lipoma) and inflammatory lesions and directing the veterinarian to perform further tests on lesions that may be cancerous. In some patients, cytology may be equivocal and a biopsy may be required to reach a definitive diagnosis. Cytology should be performed with the objective of answering four questions:

1. Is this neoplastic or not (e.g., inflammatory)?
2. If neoplastic, does it look benign or malignant?
3. If malignant, what type of cell is involved (epithelial (carcinoma), mesenchymal (sarcoma) or round cell tumor?
4. Are there characteristics that can allow a diagnosis (i.e., osteosarcoma, lymphoma, mast cell tumor)?

In reality, the first of these four steps may be the only important one in clinical practice, and the last three are really for a trained cytopathologist to decide. If the first step shows it to be suggestive of neoplasia, a biopsy is indicated.

The most common method of collecting a cytology specimen is by fine-needle aspiration cytology. Fine-needle aspiration (FNA) cytology can be used to screen primary lesions for the presence of cancer, or in the staging process (see Chapter 4) to determine whether lymph nodes or other secondary sites are involved with cancer. Fine-needle aspiration cytology uses a fine-gauge (22 or 23) needle on a syringe, usually 5 ml, and preferably not Luer-Lok. Slides are cleaned and laid out before the sampling is done. The needle is attached to the syringe and directed into the lesion, and suction is applied to the syringe several times to draw cells into the barrel of the needle. Pressure should be sufficient to draw cells into the hub of the needle, but not so much that the sample is drawn into the syringe, because this would usually be contaminated with blood (Figure 3.1).

Suction is then let off the syringe to allow cells to remain in the barrel of the needle and not be aspirated into the syringe, and the needle is withdrawn from the lesion. The needle is then detached from the syringe, and the syringe is filled with air and then reattached. The sample is then blown out of the needle and onto the slide by expelling air from the syringe through the needle (Figure 3.2). Depending on the consistency of the sample, it will usually need to be smeared on the slide using a procedure similar to making a blood smear (Figure 3.3).

A second FNA technique is the "needle-off" collection technique. In this method, the needle alone is introduced into the lesion and moved in and out, slightly altering the angle each time. After 5 to 10 passes, the needle is withdrawn and attached to an air-filled syringe. From this point, sample handling is the same as outlined above. There is no absolute advantage to either method, but rather the choice should be directed by the individual tumor and patient characteristics.

A third method of making cytology slides from a piece of tissue is by making "touch" preparations. This is often done when a biopsy sample has been collected, and cytologic evaluation will allow a quicker preliminary result while the histopathology is pending. By this technique the sample is gently blotted to remove any clots or excessive blood. It is then touched to a clean, dry glass slide to make an imprint. This is repeated for small

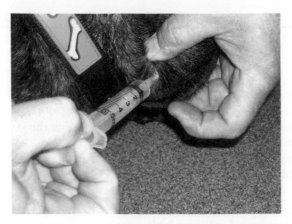

**Figure 3.1.** This illustrates the positioning for aspiration from the mandibular lymph node of a dog with suspected metastatic mast cell tumor. The needle is repositioned while keeping mild negative pressure sufficient to pull material into the needle hub, but not so much that it enters the syringe where the sample may be contaminated by blood (making interpretation more difficult).

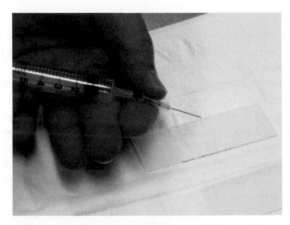

**Figure 3.2.** The cytology sample is expelled onto a clean glass slide by disconnecting the needle from the syringe, filling the syringe with air and reattaching, and then pushing the air out through the needle to "blow" cells onto the slide.

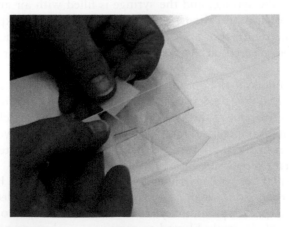

**Figure 3.3.** The sample is then gently prepared as for a blood smear, by gently placing a slide on top of the sample and pulling them apart without downward pressure (that will rupture the cells).

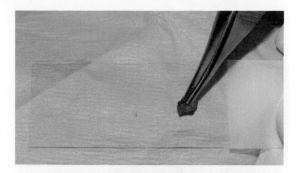

**Figure 3.4.** For impression smears, the sample is blotted gently to remove blood and then "prints" are made on the clean glass slide.

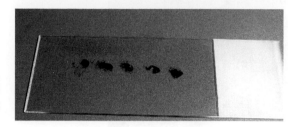

**Figure 3.5.** Impression smears (here stained) can provide an excellent preparation for cytology and may allow earlier preliminary results while waiting for results of histopathology.

samples until there are 4 or 5 "touch-prints" on the slide (see Figures 3.4 and 3.5). After touch preparations are made, the tissue sample can then be placed in fixative.

Whatever method is used, slides are then dried and left unstained for submission to a reference laboratory; if they are to be assessed in-house, they can be stained using a commercially available 3-step quick stain. The staining process is as follows:

1.  Once you have the slides with the cytology specimen, ensure it is completely dry. This can be achieved by either moving it gently through the air (don't drop it); or by running a gentle, low-heat, hair dryer over the slide.
2.  The dried slide is place in the fixative (solution 1), and left to fix for 1 minute.
3.  Without rinsing, transfer the slide to solution 2 (red) and "swish" the slide through the solution for 15 swishes.
4.  Blot the excess red solution 2 from the bottom edge of the slide, and then
5.  Without rinsing, transfer the slide to solution 3 (purple) and "swish" the slide through the solution for 15 swishes.
6.  Rinse gently under running water and air dry for microscopic evaluation.

If the staining is not intense enough (e.g., in some mast cell tumors the granules may be difficult to see), additional "swishes" in purple can be done even if it is dried (as long as there is no immersion oil on the slide).

## Tumor Histopathology

Although it is more expensive and time-consuming to perform a biopsy and histopathology, in many cases it is the only way to obtain a definitive diagnosis on a particular tumor.

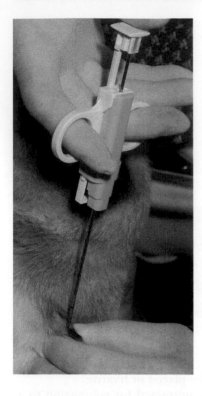

**Figure 3.6.** The technique of obtaining a Tru-cut needle core sample from a subcutaneous mass on a dog. (Courtesy of Dr. Gregory K. Ogilvie)

The main types of biopsy are needle core biopsy (Tru-cut biopsy), which is done using a large needle that cuts a core of tissue (Figure 3.6), and surgical biopsy. Surgical biopsy may be either incisional, where a small piece of tumor tissue is removed for analysis, or excisional, where the entire lesion is removed and submitted. Biopsy is usually performed under general anesthesia and requires careful planning so as not to negatively impact future definitive surgery or radiotherapy. Biopsy is safe and, despite some commonly held beliefs and anecdotes, it does not contribute to tumor metastasis. Metastasis is a complex biologic process that involves multiple phenotypic alterations in cancer cells; not a simple matter of access to the bloodstream.

It is extremely important that any samples submitted for histopathological examination are representative of the lesion (this is the veterinarian's task) and that they are collected and handled carefully to avoid crush artifacts (particularly of small biopsies) prior to placing in formalin fixative. The veterinary cancer nurse can help by learning techniques for gentle handling of needle core biopsy samples (Figure 3.7) and always picking up smaller biopsy samples with gloved fingers, with a needle, or with rat's-tooth forceps to avoid crushing the delicate margins. If a sample must be stored temporarily prior to placing in fixative, it should be placed in a saline-moistened gauze pad until ready.

Endoscopy samples are very small, and they are best handled with a fine-gauge needle (Figure 3.8). The needle can be used to transfer the sample to a plastic cassette that will hold them in place while in the fixative (Figure 3.9). This technique also makes it easier for the pathologist to identify the samples and prevents them from clumping together.

The technician should always check how the sample needs to be fixed, and whether any other evaluations should be done before placing the biopsy in formalin. Other fixatives (Z-fix, ethanol) may be preferred for specimens destined for immunohistochemical "special"

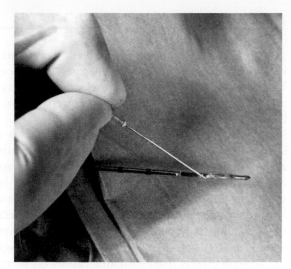

**Figure 3.7.** A small-gauge needle is used to gently lift the sample from the biopsy needle (maintain sterility so the biopsy needle can be used to obtain further samples). It can then be placed in fixative. Some pathologists prefer the sample to be placed in a plastic cassette or on a card to maintain the structure of the sample.

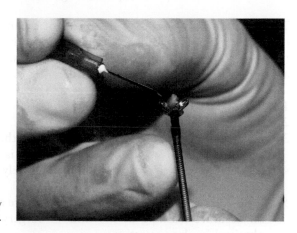

**Figure 3.8.** Use a fine gauge needle to gently remove an endoscopy sample from the biopsy cup.

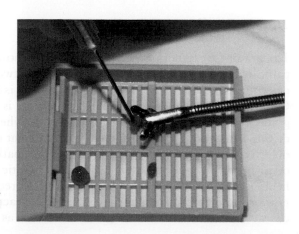

**Figure 3.9.** The needle is used to place samples on a plastic cassette for easy identification and separation during fixation.

stains. Also, once in formalin, cytologic examination is no longer possible due to alteration in the appearance of the cells. In some cases, a cytological evaluation can be done with biopsy samples to provide a quicker preliminary result while the biopsy is pending, by making a series of "touch" cytology preparations (above under "Cytology"), but this can be done only before fixation.

Always ensure that the volume of fixative is adequate for the biopsy sample that is immersed in it (i.e., 10 volumes of formalin fixative to 1 volume of tissue specimen). Also avoid "jamming" large tissue specimens into narrow-neck containers. For larger specimens check with your lab personnel because they may be able to provide you with appropriately sized containers. It may also improve the speed and completeness of fixation (which translates into faster more accurate results), if the specimen is sliced (like a loaf of bread) prior to immersing it in fixative. If cytological specimens are to be submitted together with histopathology specimens, ensure that the cytology slides are "bagged" separately to avoid the adverse effects from formalin vapors on them.

## What a Veterinary Histopathologist Can Provide

The selection and success of treatment of a cancer patient is directly dependent on the information obtained from a veterinary histopathologist. As long as there is adequate tissue of a representative nature available for review, the histopathologist should be able to answer such questions as the following:

1. Is it neoplastic/cancerous?
2. What type of tumor is it?
3. Has the tumor metastasized (depending on the tissue sampled) or is there blood vessel and lymphatic invasion that could mean it is likely to metastasize?
4. Is the tumor likely to have been completely excised (if the entire excised tissue is submitted)?
5. If the tumor is not completely excised, where are the margins closest (this may depend on accurate marking at the time of surgery) and what margin (in mm) has been obtained in close resections.
6. Would additional stains or tests allow better characterization of this tumor?

## Tumor Grading and Staging

The grading of tumors is perhaps one of the most important tasks of a veterinary histopathologist. There is often some confusion between the term *grade*, which is primarily determined by histopathology, and *stage*, which is primarily determined clinically (see also Chapter 4). The biological behavior of tumors is not always predicted by the histologic grade; however, there is a long list of tumors where grade is extremely important in predicting behavior and hence in directing treatment options. Grading is performed by either objective or subjective evaluation of the histopathologic characteristics of cancer and is often based on mitotic index (number of mitotic figures per 10 high-power microscope fields (hpf)), the degree of differentiation, degree of cellular or nuclear pleomorphism, proportion of necrosis, invasiveness, stromal reaction, and inflammatory response. These characteristics can be used to grade the tumor as a low-grade (well-differentiated, grade

1), intermediate grade (moderately differentiated, grade 2), or high-grade (poorly differentiated, grade 3) tumor. Grading does include some subjective criteria; therefore, variation may occur between pathologists when an individual tumor is graded. Providing complete clinical information, and the largest and best quality sample possible, can help.

Examples where grade is an important prognostic factor include mast cell tumors, soft tissue sarcomas, melanoma, mammary gland carcinoma, synovial cell sarcoma, multilobular osteochondrosarcoma, hemangiosarcoma, splenic sarcomas, transitional cell carcinoma, squamous cell carcinoma, pulmonary carcinoma, osteosarcoma, histiocytic sarcomas, and lymphoma.

The histopathologist may further assist in *staging* the tumor by determining the size of the tumor (measurement of the tumor specimen submitted), depth of invasion into surrounding normal tissues and by identification of blood or lymphatic vessel invasion by tumor emboli, or of metastasis to regional lymph nodes or other distant sites, such as the lung. Like grading, staging is essential to direct therapy and to help render an accurate prognosis.

## Evaluation of Tumor Margins

For surgery to be successful, complete margins of normal tissue around the tumor are essential whether the tumor is benign or malignant. Margins should be checked in all directions including those lateral and deep to the tumor, and this can be done only if all resected tissue is submitted for histopathology. This process can be made more helpful to the cancer treatment team if different colored inks or sutures are placed to guide the pathologist to the particular areas that the surgeon feels the least "comfortable" about having removed with adequate margins (Figures 3.10 and 3.11). A note should be made in the patient's record as to the stain and anatomic location, for example "blue = caudal margin; black = deep margin."

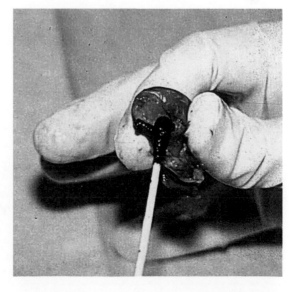

**Figure 3.10.** India ink, or a commercial colored ink preparation, is used to identify edges of the tissue surrounding a tumor where surgeons are concerned about their ability to completely excise the cancer. Multiple colored inks allow multiple margins to be identified and correlated with anatomic positioning. This can be helpful if further surgery needs to be planned. (Courtesy of Dr. Robert McCarthy)

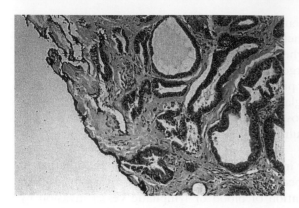

**Figure 3.11.** This is how the pathologist views the slide. You can see that the inked margin is clearly visible, allowing the pathologist to evaluate completeness of surgical excision. (Courtesy of Dr. Robert McCarthy)

## Special Stains

Although the diagnosis of cancer still relies heavily on morphologic assessment of specimens under light microscopy with routine staining (hematoxylin and eosin; H & E), in some situations, the tumors may be too poorly differentiated to determine their cell of origin. The use of special stains can be helpful in determining the tissue of origin, which can be pivotal for treatment and hence outcome.

Immunohistochemistry is a specialized area of cancer pathology where staining antibodies are directed toward specific epitopes such as intermediate filaments, secretory substances, hormones, and proteins of various types. Immunohistochemistry takes advantage of the preservation of certain molecules that can demonstrate the cell of origin of an otherwise undifferentiated neoplasm.

# Staging of Cancer 4

Each tumor and patient is different. When evaluating a pet for treatment of cancer it is important not only to obtain a definitive histologic diagnosis and, where appropriate, a grade determined by an experienced, specially trained histopathologist (see Chapter 3), but also to perform staging. Staging is sometimes confused with *grading* (an assessment of the histopathologic features of the tumor assigned by the pathologist). *Staging* is a clinical process that enables us to evaluate the pet's general health, identifying unrelated or secondary conditions that need to be treated or controlled before instituting appropriate therapy, and to quantitate the extent of cancer involvement in the patient. The prognostic information gained by doing this is important in order to make informed and rational decisions as to the type of therapy best suited for the individual patient. Thus, the staging process is an essential component of pretreatment care to maximize effective treatment and minimize toxicity.

## The TNM System

The exact staging system varies with different tumor types, and these are generally established by the World Health Organization (WHO). Most staging systems for solid (nonhematologic) tumors are based an assessment of three major components of the malignant process:

1. The size of the primary tumor (T)
2. The presence and extent of lymph node metastasis (N)
3. And the presence of distant metastasis (M)

These components are further modified by the use of subscript numbers to indicate increasing tumor size, progressive involvement of regional lymph nodes, and other modifiers depending on the particular tumor.

Although the specific staging scheme varies among tumor types, in general the process begins with a thorough physical examination to identify any enlarged lymph nodes or other obvious areas of cancer involvement, a complete blood count, chemistry profile, urinalysis, thoracic radiographs (both right and left laterals plus either a ventrodorsal or dorsoventral view), and abdominal radiographs or ultrasonography. In addition, ancillary diagnostics such as cardiac ultrasonography, computerized tomography, magnetic resonance imaging, or other more specialized tests may be required.

## Staging and Health

The staging process also evaluates the general health of the patient. Cancer patients are often geriatric and may have the potential for a number of underlying conditions that may adversely affect their health and the potential success of therapy. Also, any neoplastic process may result in a number of paraneoplastic conditions that affect the well-being of the cancer patient. In addition, other unrelated but serious concerns may be identified that may bear on the patient's overall prognosis and could affect decisions regarding treatment options.

In many instances, correcting or supporting underlying problems such as renal failure, urinary tract infections, heart disease, and metabolic disturbances may significantly improve the general health of the patient and thus improve the potential for successful cancer care, as well as the patient's overall quality of life.

When complicated surgical procedures or multiple radiation therapies that require repeated or prolonged anesthesia are planned, adequate renal and hepatic functions are vital.

The likelihood of a successful outcome for a patient treated with chemotherapy is as dependent on drug metabolism and elimination (and drug absorption for orally administered chemotherapy) as it is on the sensitivity of the tumor. Consequently, information gained during staging may identify problems that will impact the type and dosage of chemotherapy to optimize efficacy while limiting toxicity.

For example, hepatic dysfunction may lead to delayed chemotherapy elimination (examples; vinca alkaloids, doxorubicin) and therefore to greater toxicity such as myelosuppression. In contrast, cyclophosphamide is activated in the liver so hepatic dysfunction may result in poor efficacy.

Similarly, renal dysfunction may worsen toxicity for some drugs that are themselves nephrotoxic. For example, cisplatin should not be used in patients with renal azotemia. On the other hand, carboplatin is not nephrotoxic, but reduced renal excretion of carboplatin will exacerbate myelosuppression.

Particularly for those breeds with a predisposition to develop cardiomyopathy, treatment with doxorubicin should be preceded by cardiac evaluation. Pretreatment echocardiography should be performed and dogs with reduction in contractility should not receive doxorubicin. While valvular dysfunction itself is not worsened by doxorubicin and therefore is not necessarily a reason to withhold doxorubicin, it should be remembered that mild changes in cardiac muscle function may exacerbate the clinical impact of valvular disease. In these patients, echocardiography should be performed periodically through treatment, ideally prior to each treatment. Treatment should be discontinued if contractility is below normal, and while the patient is still asymptomatic. Cardiac dysfunction due to doxorubicin is irreversible and usually progressive. For this reason, waiting until the patient has signs of early cardiac failure before discontinuing doxorubicin is unacceptable practice.

## Reevaluation

During and after a course of treatment, restaging is sometimes required. The most common reason for this is to assess a patients' response to treatment. However patients may also need to be restaged to reevaluate the extent of disease and general health at the time of relapse or recurrence prior to restarting treatment.

## Staging Tests

The following sections summarize some common assessments used in the staging process.

### *Physical Examination*

The physical examination is critical in staging any tumor, as well as establishing some prognostic criteria. Two of the most important pieces of information gained from the physical examination are tumor size and location. For various tumors, these factors may hold important prognostic significance. For almost any solid tumor, they are important factors to consider with regard to the potential for local therapy. Physical examination is also an important tool for screening for other health problems (unrelated or paraneoplastic) that may affect the patient's treatment or prognosis.

Physical examination is easy to perform and minimally invasive, and it provides critical information for staging and prognosis. Physical examination findings will often direct the clinician to further testing that is needed (imaging, biopsy, and so forth).

A set of calipers that measure in millimeters is extremely useful. Tumor size should be measured using calipers and the longest dimension, the greatest width, and the maximum depth recorded at each visit (Figure 4.1). The veterinary cancer nurse can assist by making sure that accurate measurements are included in the permanent record for the patient. Table 4.1 is a suggested format for lymph node measurements. This can be critical to assessing treatment response and prognosis. For example, if a dog with lymphoma has large lymph nodes a week after chemotherapy, and the original measurements are not recorded, does this mean it is progressing (poor prognosis, requires a change of treatment), or that it has responded partially but not completely (much more encouraging and treatment should be continued).

### *Complete Blood Count*

A complete blood count (CBC) is always recommended for baseline staging of any pet with cancer, particularly if surgery or chemotherapy is planned. This is especially true for patients at high risk for paraneoplastic syndromes or bone marrow disease. A CBC is easy to perform and minimally invasive, and it provides critical information for planning treatment.

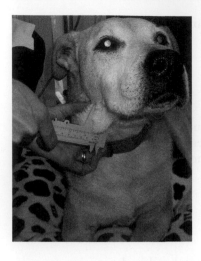

**Figure 4.1.** Calipers should be used to measure the size of tumors or lymph nodes in at least two, perpendicular dimensions. Usually the largest two diameters are measured. The results should be recorded in the patient's medical record in a chart format (see Table 4.1).

**Table 4.1.** Example of a table used to keep lymph node measurements

| Patient Name | | Date | |
| --- | --- | --- | --- |
| Lymph Node | Measurements in Millimeters | Measurements in Millimeters | |
| **Mandibular** | | | |
| **Prescapular** | | | |
| **Axillary** | | | |
| **Popliteal** | | | |
| **Inguinal** | | | |
| **Other** | | | |

Hematologic evaluation is an important part of initial diagnostics and staging in cancer patients, as well as a vital part of ongoing monitoring for patients undergoing treatment. The cancer process may cause hematologic abnormalities either by direct involvement of the bone marrow or via paraneoplastic effects; these may provide clues that can aid the diagnostic process or require management themselves. Another reason to be aware of the patient's baseline CBC results is that during cancer treatment, some of the most common side effects of chemotherapy are hematologic.

Many cancer patients have anemia detected on baseline CBC evaluations. Potential causes can include anemia of chronic disease, blood loss, immune-mediated hemolytic anemia, and marrow infiltration by disease.

Anemia of chronic disease occurs when red blood cell lifespan is shortened, compounded by disordered iron metabolism and blunted erythropoietin response. This is usually a low-grade, normocytic, normochromic, and nonregenerative anemia. It is not usually a significant clinical problem and usually resolves (sometimes slowly) with tumor control.

Acute blood loss can result in a regenerative anemia; if very recent, the anemia may appear nonregenerative. Chronic blood loss results in a microcytic (low MCV), hypochromic (low MCHC) anemia. Common sites of bleeding include splenic or hepatic tumors, nasal tumors, and GI tumors. Even if not involved in tumor, the GI tract may also be a site of blood loss as a paraneoplastic effect in mast cell tumors and gastrinomas.

Immune-mediated hemolytic anemia can occur as a paraneoplastic effect in a number of cancers, particularly lymphoma. This anemia varies in severity, is usually regenerative, and can be acute or chronic.

Primary erythrocytosis, or polycythemia vera, is a myeloproliferative disorder of the erythroid lines that results in an elevated red cell count and is treated as a leukemia. Secondary erythrocytosis can be seen as a rare paraneoplastic syndrome associated mostly with renal tumors, but other tumors have also been reported to result in this condition.

Leukemias can result in increased numbers of any line of circulating cells, the most common in dogs and cats being lymphoid leukemias. Increased circulating lymphoid cells can also occur with stage 5 lymphoma. In chronic leukemias the circulating cells may resemble normal cells cytologically. Increased circulating numbers of white blood cells can also occur as paraneoplastic syndromes, and it is necessary to differentiate a chronic leukemia from a paraneoplastic syndrome.

Decreased numbers of white blood cells usually raise a suspicion of bone marrow infiltration with cancer (myelophthisis), particularly if multiple blood cell types are affected. Pancytopenia (reduced numbers of multiple types of blood cells) is most commonly caused by leukemia, but it can also occur as a paraneoplastic syndrome with estrogen-producing tumors (Sertoli cell tumors), which may not resolve, even with removal of the tumor.

Thrombocytopenia can occur as a result of several mechanisms, including myelophthisis, immune-mediated destruction, and consumption. Thrombocytosis can occur as a rare paraneoplastic syndrome or as part of a reactive process.

Chapter 13 presents detail on interpreting hematologic changes and hematologic supportive care, especially in patients undergoing chemotherapy.

## Serum Biochemistry Panel

A full serum chemistry panel is always recommended for baseline staging of any pet with cancer, particularly if surgery, chemotherapy, or multiple anesthesias (such as for radiotherapy) are anticipated. This is even more critical for geriatric patients or those at high risk for paraneoplastic syndromes (e.g., dogs with lymphoma). Information gained from these evaluations can also be helpful in planning for supportive and palliative care. These tests are easy to perform, relatively reliable, and minimally invasive. Findings that may be relevant in evaluation of a cancer patient and treatment planning can include those discussed in the following sections.

### Alanine Aminotransferase (ALT)

In dogs with ALT elevations, measurement of bile acids (see the section "Ancillary Blood and Urine Testing" later in this chapter) is a more specific test for hepatic dysfunction, which can affect chemotherapy drug metabolism and result in altered toxicity (see also "Bilirubin," below).

Some chemotherapeutics are hepatotoxic. Dogs with elevated ALT prior to receiving a dose of CCNU are at increased risk of toxicity. Also, CCNU may cause elevations in serum ALT activity prior to causing functional hepatopathy, and prompt discontinuation of the drug when the ALT rises will resolve the problem in most dogs before it becomes a clinical toxicity. Therefore, monitoring of serum ALT prior to patients receiving each dose of CCNU is a good screening test for toxicity.

## Alkaline Phosphatase (ALP)

Multiple studies have demonstrated an association between elevated serum alkaline phosphatase (ALP) activity at the time of diagnosis and poor survival after amputation for osteosarcoma. In one of these, elevated serum total ALP levels were associated with a shorter survival time of 5.5 months, versus 12.5 months for dogs with normal serum ALP. Serum bone-ALP levels may be even more powerful in their ability to predict survival in dogs with osteosarcoma.

## Bilirubin

Monitoring the bilirubin level is important when hepatically metabolized or hepatotoxic drugs are to be used. An elevated bilirubin levels indicate much more advanced hepatic damage than do elevated hepatocellular enzyme (e.g., ALT) levels. Chemotherapy drugs that are metabolized by the liver (e.g., vincristine, vinblastine, and doxorubicin) will cause exaggerated toxicity if administered to a patient with liver dysfunction; therefore, doses of these drugs should be reduced for patients with liver dysfunction.

## Creatinine

Elevated serum creatinine, if accompanied by isosthenuria or hyposthenuria, is indicative of renal dysfunction. When the urine specific gravity is high, an elevated creatinine level suggests dehydration. In older cats, serum creatinine should also be interpreted in light of serum T4 level; i.e., hyperthyroidism may mask renal insufficiency. In animals with renal dysfunction, doses of renally excreted chemotherapy drugs (e.g., carboplatin) should be reduced, and nephrotoxic drugs (e.g., cisplatin in dogs and doxorubicin in cats) should be avoided altogether.

## Urea

Elevated urea with a normal creatinine and urine specific gravity can occur with a high protein diet, but in other patients it may be suggestive of GI tract hemorrhage, so this possibility should be considered in light of the clinical history (mast cell tumor, NSAID therapy, etc.).

## Calcium

Hypercalcemia is one of the most common paraneoplastic syndromes seen in veterinary oncology (see Chapter 19, "Metabolic Emergencies," for emergency management of hypercalcemia). When it occurs it is most commonly associated with lymphoid malignancies or anal sac adenocarcinoma but has less commonly been associated with many other cancer types. Occasionally the PU/PD caused by hypercalcemia is the first presenting sign of one of these cancers. Severe hypercalcemia requires immediate management to avoid the development of hypercalcemic nephropathy and permanent renal failure. The serum calcium level should always be interpreted in light of the serum albumin level.

## Albumin

Increased albumin concentration should prompt consideration of dehydration. Decreased albumin can occur with various metabolic abnormalities including liver failure, renal disease, hemorrhage, and GI tract disease (maldigestion, malabsorption). Decreased albumin concentration can affect other tests (i.e., hypoalbuminemia artifactually decreases the calcium level) and drug binding.

## Globulin

Hyperglobulinemia may be polyclonal or monoclonal, and serum protein electrophoresis is necessary to make this critical distinction. When polyclonal, the most likely cause is chronic inflammation/infectious disease, although less commonly a polyclonal gammopathy can be associated with cancer. When monoclonal (or biclonal) gammopathy is identified. The most common cause is plasma cell cancer (often known as *multiple myeloma*); however, other malignancies and even infectious disease (e.g., *Ehrlichiosis*) can less commonly be a cause.

## Glucose

Hypoglycemia is seen as a paraneoplastic syndrome with a variety of neoplasms, including large hepatic tumors and insulinomas (see Chapter 19 for emergency management of hypoglycemia). Abdominal ultrasonography and measurement of serum insulin level should be considered.

## *Urine Evaluation*

Urinalysis is a commonly overlooked test in patients not displaying signs referable to the urinary tract. However, it is an important part of pretreatment baseline evaluation in cancer patients. Urinalysis allows more accurate evaluation of renal function, which can be important in anticipating toxicity because many drugs are renally excreted. The urine specific gravity is important in interpreting changes in urea and creatinine (see above). Presence of proteinuria may elucidate a finding of hypoalbuminemia. However, Bence-Jones proteinuria (light chain globulin fragments in the urine, as seen in myeloma-related disorders) is not detectable on routine urinalysis.

Secondary urinary tract infections can particularly occur in animals with urinary tract tumors or hemorrhagic cystitis as a chemotherapy side effect, and the diagnosis of an infection does not rule out these possibilities as an underlying cause. In addition, pets with many types of cancer may be immunosuppressed and will have a "clinically silent" urinary tract infection. Such an infection can worsen, and/or act as a source for sepsis if a myelosuppressive chemotherapy drug is given. Concurrent treatment of the infection based on culture and sensitivity will allow chemotherapy to be given while reducing the risk of life-threatening sepsis.

## Lymph Node Evaluation

For many cancers, the first site of metastasis may be the draining (regional) lymph nodes. At diagnosis, all lymph nodes should be carefully palpated, with special attention to those draining the primary tumor (see Figure 4.1). For inguinal or perineal tumors, the draining lymph nodes are evaluated by abdominal ultrasonography. Enlarged or firm nodes should be further evaluated by fine-needle aspiration cytology, and cytology that is suspicious but not definitive should be confirmed by surgical biopsy. For some cancers, the lymph node metastatic rate is so high that even normal-size lymph nodes should be aspirated or biopsied.

Fine-needle aspiration of peripheral lymph nodes is easy to perform and minimally invasive, and it provides important staging information (see Chapter 3). For intraabdominal nodes the process is more involved but generally not insurmountable if ultrasonography is available. As discussed above, cytology results are sometimes equivocal and may require biopsy for confirmation.

## Imaging

### Radiography

X-rays are absorbed in the body according to the density of the material they pass through, so materials such as bone or metal allow less energy to reach the film and the image is white; whereas air is less dense, more energy is transmitted and the image is blacker. Therefore, radiographs are especially suited for disclosing changes to bone and lungs and to tissue and organ boundaries, whereas soft tissue and parenchymal changes (such as within the liver, spleen, or kidneys) are more difficult to visualize. Radiographs can be taken safely and the necessary equipment is widely available. Sedation may be required for appropriate positioning. Specific training is needed to obtain good quality radiographs (technician's role) and for interpretation of the images (veterinarian's role). Appropriate protective measures must be taken to minimize the risk of radiation exposure.

Thoracic radiographs may disclose pulmonary metastasis (Figure 4.2), and concurrent diseases may also be found, especially in geriatric patients. Good quality three-view (both laterals as well as ventrodorsal or dorsoventral) thoracic radiographs should be performed for patients with any cancer that has a risk of pulmonary metastasis or intrathoracic spread. Pulmonary metastases may be visible on one lateral view but not the other (Figures 4.3 and 4.4).

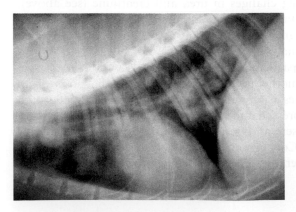

**Figure 4.2.** Metastatic hemangiosarcoma in a cat; the multiple nodular densities in the thoracic radiograph are typical for carcinoma and sarcoma metastases.

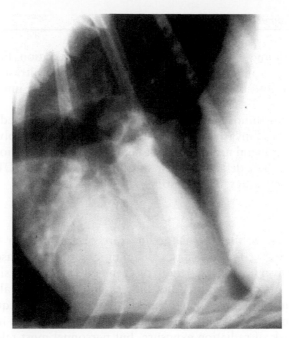

**Figure 4.3.** A right lateral radiograph of a dog with systemic histiocytic sarcoma. The appearance was considered normal. (Courtesy of Dr. Kenneth M. Rassnick)

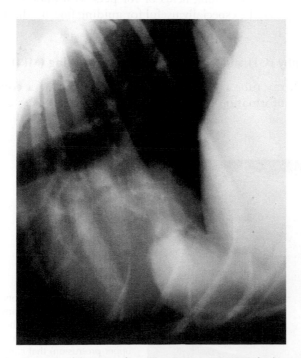

**Figure 4.4.** A left lateral radiograph of the same dog seen in Figure 4.3. Note the large caudoventral pulmonary mass that was not visible on the other view. (Courtesy of Dr. Kenneth M. Rassnick)

Abdominal radiography may confirm a physical examination finding of probable abdominal mass and may indicate its location; but abdominal ultrasonography provides information about the internal organ architecture (liver, kidneys, intestinal tract) and is preferred.

For a musculoskeletal tumor, fine detail radiographs of the affected area may provide information on its size and invasiveness, particularly if the tumor involves bone. However, more than 50% of the mineral needs to be lost before osteolysis is radiographically visible, so plain radiographs do not definitively rule out bone damage, and CT scanning or MRI should be considered to address this question.

### Ultrasonography

Ultrasonography can image the internal architecture of an organ or tumor, which may prove valuable in assessing for metastases or guiding surgery. Ultrasonography is safe, painless, and noninvasive; however sedation, or even general anaesthesia (for guided biopsies), may be needed. Access is required not only to equipment, but also to the expertise for interpretation of ultrasound imaging; considerable expertise is required to accurately interpret ultrasound images especially to do so reproducibly for repeat imaging in the same patient. There is no risk of radiation exposure, but personnel must take appropriate precautions to protect themselves from repetitive strain injury.

Most intraabdominal tumors are better imaged by ultrasonography than by radiographs. Some cancers (e.g., splenic hemangiosarcoma) are likely to metastasize to intraabdominal sites, and for these, abdominal ultrasonography is an important part of staging and restaging (Figure 4.5).

For a mass at the periphery of lung fields or for pets with abdominal or thoracic effusions, ultrasonography may be especially useful for guiding fine-needle aspiration or needle biopsy.

### Computed Tomography (CT) and Magnetic Resonance Imaging (MRI)

In CT scanning an X-ray tube rotates around the patient while a computer collects the results and from this information creates images called *slices*. Slices can be studied indi-

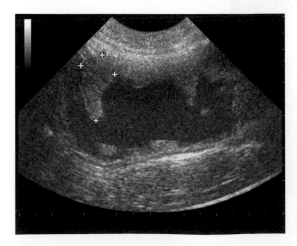

**Figure 4.5.** An ultrasonogram of the urinary bladder of a dog with transitional cell carcinoma. Multiple protrusions of the tumor are visible, and accurate measurements can be obtained (see left upper protrusion) that can be used to measure the efficacy of treatment in causing tumor response ("restaging").

vidually or placed together to form a three-dimensional image of the area of the patient being studied.

MRI scanning uses magnets and radio waves to create the images, producing images that have much higher soft tissue detail.

Although they are painless and noninvasive, CT and MRI scanning both require general anesthesia to immobilize veterinary patients in the machine (which can be anxiety-provoking in human patients). In addition, because CT scanning uses X-rays, appropriate measures must be taken to protect personnel from the risk of radiation exposure. Both CT and MRI are relatively costly compared to radiography and ultrasonography; access is required to both equipment and special expertise for interpretation of images. If radiotherapy or extensive surgery are being considered, the surgeon or radiation oncologist that will be performing the treatment should be consulted prior to CT or MRI to ensure that correct views are obtained.

When thoracic radiographs are equivocal for pulmonary metastasis, thoracic CT scanning is often able to confirm or deny the presence of even small (3 mm) pulmonary nodules.

Abdominal ultrasonography is an important part of staging for many intraabdominal cancers, but CT scanning can provide even more objective images and measurements, and it can be used with contrast imaging to highlight equivocal tumors or to delineate margins around invasive tumors (Figures 4.6 and 4.7).

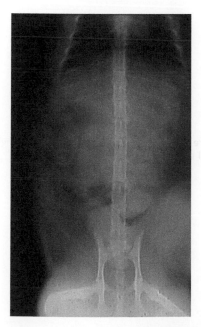

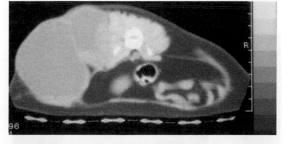

**Figure 4.6.** An abdominal radiograph of a cat with an injection site sarcoma over the left hip area. On radiographs the soft tissue density is readily apparent, but the margins are not. Both surgery and radiotherapy are options for this patient, but without knowing the extent of the tumor, an accurate prognosis is difficult.

**Figure 4.7.** A CT image slice from the same cat in Figure 4.6. The extent of the tumor and invasion around the spine means that surgery alone is unlikely to provide good tumor control. The field for radiotherapy can now be accurately set, using the CT image. In addition, the risk of radiation toxicity to underlying organs can be assessed and hopefully avoided.

Because mineral loss must be extensive before it is radiographically visible, CT scanning is far more accurate for delineation of tumor extent in bone, and it should be considered if the tumor margins are uncertain or if radiation therapy or a challenging surgery is being considered. This is particularly true of tumors involving the head and neck or pelvic region. MRI is best used when soft-tissue detail is needed, such as spine, brain, or muscle.

Naturally, using these modalities will not be able to guarantee that a tumor can be completely eradicated by radiation or surgery; however, it will certainly improve the likelihood by enabling better planning of surgical approach or radiation field, and it may prevent a needless attempt at a treatment that can not be successful because of tumor extent or location.

CT and MRI may be helpful in restaging of patients to assess the response to chemotherapy or radiotherapy, and to decide whether further therapy is indicated (Figures 4.8–4.11).

CT scans can also be used to create 3-D images that allow a surgeon to plan surgery, and a radiation oncologist to protect normal surrounding tissues, by adjusting the dose beam. CT scans also enable owners to more clearly visualize the tumor and conceptualize what will happen to their pet (Figures 4.12 and 4.13).

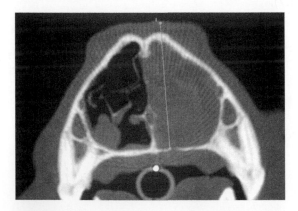

**Figure 4.8.** A CT scan from a dog with a right-sided nasal carcinoma before radiotherapy.

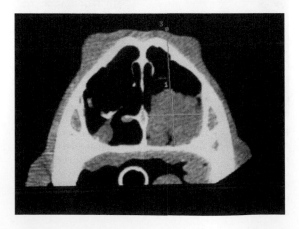

**Figure 4.9.** A CT scan slice from the same level on the dog seen in Figure 4.8, but 3 months after radiotherapy. There is clearly tumor response in this restaging scan.

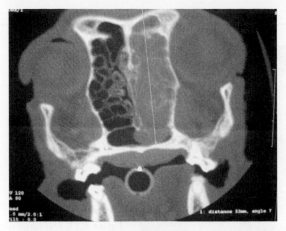

**Figure 4.10.** A CT scan from the dog seen in Figure 4.8, at another slice level, before radiotherapy.

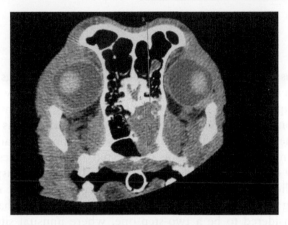

**Figure 4.11.** The same slice level as seen in Figure 4.10, but again, 3 months after treatment, clearly showing response. Future imaging can be considered to assess the patient if there are signs that could signal tumor growth or infection. CT scans with baseline information can help distinguish between these possibilities.

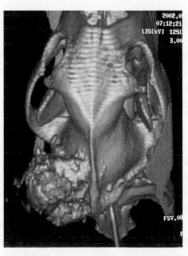

**Figure 4.12.** A CT reconstruction of a multilobular osteochondrosarcoma (MLO) of the base of the skull. Such an image is very powerful when explaining treatment options to an owner. (Courtesy of Dr. David Simpson)

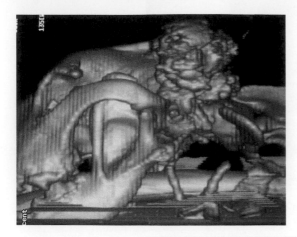

**Figure 4.13.** The same dog as seen in Figure 4.12, from a lateral view. (Courtesy of Dr. David Simpson)

## Bone Scintigraphy

Most of the studies using bone scintigraphy (technetium scans) in dogs with bone tumors, have been as a screen to see whether they have additional bony sites when they have been diagnosed with an appendicular osteosarcoma. Under these circumstances, one of the drawbacks is that bone scintigraphy may detect other lesions, such as osteoarthritis both in bone and soft tissue sites. In one group of 66 dogs with appendicular osteosarcoma that underwent technetium scintigraphy, none manifested other bony lesions. However, in another series of 399 dogs, in 7.8% of cases scintigraphy detected suspicious lesions that also appeared on radiographs and were metastatic sites, but yet were not suspected clinically (i.e., not causing lameness or pain). Bone scintigraphy does not have high resolution, so the process is considered to be a two-step one, where unusual sites of bone activity would be further imaged by radiographs or CT or MRI after radioactivity is back to normal levels.

## Ancillary Blood and Urine Testing

In cancer patients, basic testing such as CBC, biochemistry panel, and urinalysis are a vital component of diagnostics and the best possible management. However, these tests may not always give enough information for optimal patient care. In these cases, ancillary testing may be used to determine supplementary information about individual patients.

### Creatinine Clearance

Some chemotherapy agents are nephrotoxic (e.g., cisplatin and streptozotocin in dogs, doxorubicin in cats), and some are renally cleared (e.g., carboplatin). Many of our older oncology patients have renal insufficiency that may not be causing azotemia (renal function must decrease by 75% before azotemia is detected). One option for older patients with renal azotemia who require carboplatin chemotherapy is to perform an arbitrary dose reduction (25–50%). This approach may leave some animals undertreated, with a resistant tumor cell population, and others that still show marked myelosuppression. Even in animals where there is no renal azotemia, there is commonly individual variability for dosing intervals with carboplatin; some animals may take 5 or more weeks to recover to a level where a subsequent dose can be delivered safely.

Recent studies in cats have shown that basing carboplatin treatment on creatinine clearance is able to accurately direct the dose that should be used. In that study, cats that were normal, had suboptimal renal function, or were azotemic received widely ranging doses based on their creatinine clearance, but they had predictable and non–life-threatening myelosuppression. Similar strategies could be helpful in selecting carboplatin doses in dogs.

## Pre- and Postprandial Bile Acid Levels

Hepatic metabolism is important in the detoxification and excretion of many commonly used chemotherapy drugs (e.g., vincristine, vinblastine, and doxorubicin). In addition, for drugs that have hepatotoxic potential such as lomustine (CCNU), patients with any preexisting hepatic disease are at greatly increased risk of toxicity. Increases in serum hepatocellular enzyme levels should raise suspicion of hepatobiliary disease but are not specific, and other causes of such elevations may occur in both geriatric and cancer patients. In these patients, further evaluation of the liver is warranted before chemotherapy administration. Fasting serum bile acid is more specific (meaning positive is more likely to reflect true disease and less likely to give false positive), but not more sensitive (no less likely to give false negative) than serum ALP and hepatocellular enzymes levels for true hepatobiliary disease. An increased level of postprandial serum bile acid is more sensitive than is an increased level of fasting bile acids. Thus, combining fasting and postprandial bile acid levels improves both sensitivity and specificity for suspected hepatobiliary disease.

## Multiple Drug Resistance and the MDR-1 Gene

The mdr pump protein is coded for by the MDR-1 gene and is present in organs and sites such as the renal tubules, the bile ducts, and the blood brain barrier, which are important for excreting "natural toxins." It is a pump protein that crosses the cell membrane and actively removes these toxins from the cell. This protein is also present at low levels in cancer cells at the outset of chemotherapy but may increase after chemotherapy is instituted. Studies in both dogs and cats with lymphoma have found that if mdr is detected in pretreatment biopsies, the remission duration and survival times are shorter.

Some dogs have a mutation of the MDR-1 gene in their normal cells causing reduced toxin excretion, and these dogs may have reduced drug elimination and an increased tendency to toxicity. The tendency to this mutation is breed-related and is particularly well-recognized in collies, where MDR-1 mutations lead to increased sensitivity to a number of drugs, including ivermectin, but also many chemotherapeutics. Breeds that have been shown to be affected in the U.S. and Europe are collie, border collie, Shetland sheepdog, old English sheepdog, Australian shepherd, English shepherd, longhaired whippet, silken windhound, McNab, and Wäller. Affected individuals experience increased toxicity when mdr-excreted chemotherapy drugs are used. This has been shown clinically in a recent study, where affected dogs were significantly more likely to develop bone marrow suppression (neutropenia and thrombocytopenia) after vincristine chemotherapy than were dogs without mutations.

A patented test for the mutated gene is commercially available and is recommended when considering using chemotherapy to treat dogs of the breeds listed above. Dose reductions in doxorubicin, mitoxantrone, vincristine, or vinblastine (the most commonly used drugs) are recommended to avoid excess toxicity in dogs that are found to be affected.

## Veterinary Bladder Tumor Antigen (V-BTA) Test

This noninvasive urine test was developed for human patients and directed against a complex found in the urine of patients with urinary bladder transitional cell carcinoma (TCC). It has been used in humans to detect early relapse in patients treated for TCC. The test can be run using as little as 0.5 ml of urine, and it may be more accurate on centrifuged samples.

A veterinary version of the test appears to work similarly in dogs (not yet evaluated in cats). However various other urinary abnormalities increase the risk of a false positive reaction. Positive tests were seen for dogs with urinary bladder, urethral, prostatic, and even renal cancer. In studies, the sensitivity (true positive) rate is high at around 85%, and the specificity (true negative) rate is similar. For dogs with any urinary tract disease (including cancer but also other problems including simple bacterial urinary tract infection [UTI]), the specificity drops to less than 50% (meaning a high rate of false positives).

Therefore, this is not a test that can be used to detect TCC in the general population or to differentiate TCC from simple UTI in dogs showing symptoms. On the other hand, the high sensitivity means that the likelihood of missing a TCC (false negative) is very low. For this reason, the V-BTA could be used in dogs considered at high risk of developing TCC (for example, Scottish terriers, Shetland sheepdogs) as part of their geriatric wellness testing. A positive result would not tell you that the patient has TCC, but it would be a reason to investigate further. Most importantly, if the test was negative, the chances of that patient having a "silent" TCC would be very low; and the owners could feel reasonably confident that their dog was free of cancer at that time and avoid any more invasive or expensive testing.

# Further Reading

Bailey DB, et al. 2004. Effect of glomerular filtration rate on clearance and myelotoxicity of carboplatin in cats with tumors. *AJVR* 65:1502–1507.

Bergman PJ, et al. 1996. Monoclonal antibody C219 immunohistochemistry against P-glycoprotein: sequential analysis and predictive ability in dogs with lymphoma. *JVIM* 10:354–359.

Brenn SH, et al. 2008. Evaluation of P-glycoprotein expression in feline lymphoma and correlation with clinical outcome. *Vet Compar Oncol* 6:201–211.

Center SA, et al. 1990. Liver function tests in the diagnosis of portosystemic vascular anomalies. *Sem Vet Med Surg (Small Anim)* 5:94–99.

Chretin JD, et al. 2007. Reduced morbidity following prophylactic trimethoprim-sulfadiazine administration during chemotherapeutic induction: a double-blind placebo-controlled study. *JVIM* 21:141–148.

Garzotto CK, et al. 2000. Prognostic significance of serum alkaline phosphatase activity in canine appendicular osteosarcoma. *JVIM* 14:587–592.

Grindem CB, et al. 1994. Thrombocytopenia associated with neoplasia in dogs. *JVIM* 8:400–405.

Henry CJ, et al. 2003. Evaluation of a bladder tumor antigen test as a screening test for transitional cell carcinoma of the lower urinary tract in dogs. *AJVR* 64:1017–1020.

Kristal O, et al. 2004. Hepatotoxicity associated with CCNU (lomustine) chemotherapy in dogs. *JVIM* 18(1):75–80.

Lara-Garcia A, et al. 2008. Evaluation of a point-of-care hematology analyzer for use in dogs and cats receiving chemotherapeutic treatment. *JAVMA* 232(10):1488–1495.

Litster A, et al. 2007. Prevalence of bacterial species in cats with clinical signs of lower urinary tract disease: recognition of *Staphylococcus felis* as a possible feline urinary tract pathogen. *Vet Microbiol* 121:182–188.

Martinez M, et al. 2008. The pharmacogenomics of P-glycoprotein and its role in veterinary medicine. *J Vet Pharmacol Therapeutics* 31:285–300.

Mealey KL, et al. 2008. Breed distribution of the ABCB1-1 Delta (multidrug sensitivity) polymorphism among dogs undergoing ABCB1 genotyping. *JAVMA* 233:921–924.

Moore AS, et al. 2007. Doxorubicin and Bay-129566 for the treatment of osteosarcoma in dogs: A randomized, double blind, placebo controlled study. *JVIM* 21:783–790.

Webster CRL. 2005. History, clinical signs, and physical findings in hepatobiliary disease. In: Ettinger SJ, et al., eds, *Textbook of Veterinary Internal Medicine*. St Louis, Elsevier, 1422–1434.

Williams MJ, et al. 2008. Canine lymphoproliferative disease characterized by lymphocytosis: immunophenotypic markers of prognosis. *JVIM* 22:596–601.

# Section 3

## Treatment of Cancer

# General Principles of Veterinary Cancer Treatment

5

The treatment of cancer has evolved over the last few decades to parallel treatment in humans, with certain differences. The important difference between cancer therapy in humans and that offered for pet animals is in the goals of therapy. In humans, many cancers are cured, and cancer survivors may enjoy many decades of comfortable life. For this reason, treatment of cancer is aggressive and may be associated with side effects. Although pet animals are very similar biologically to humans, the chance for survival of decades is remote. Therapies are therefore directed at preserving quality of life; tumor control, or remission, is the aim rather than cure at any cost.

## Goals of Treatment

The goal of cancer treatment in human oncology is usually to cure the patient; in veterinary medicine, palliation is a more appropriate goal, and hence the drug dosages and schedules used are less likely to result in side effects. In palliative treatment the primary goal is to improve quality of life, which in veterinary medicine may result in prolonged survival because euthanasia is delayed.

Quality of life for humans depends largely on preservation of body image and essential organ function. We may interpret our impressions of a pet's well-being in terms of our own expectations and belief; communication between the cancer treatment team and the owner is therefore essential. Options for treatment should never be limited by our interpretation of the owner's finances or preferences; rather, open and honest dialogue will allow an owner to make an informed decision and will ultimately create a "team" approach to chemotherapeutic treatment of the pet's cancer. The veterinary oncology nurse is a vital part of building and maintaining that team.

The goal of veterinary cancer therapy is usually to make the pet as normal as possible with no symptoms or outward evidence of cancer. The specific treatment plan depends greatly on the tumor type. However, often the treatment starts with surgery. If the surgeon is unable to remove all the tumor cells without causing compromise to a pet's quality of life, radiation therapy may be offered as a follow-up. If the tumor has spread to other sites, or if the risk of spread is very high, treatment may involve the use of anticancer chemotherapy medications.

It is important to recognize that although cancer is a rarely curable disease, most pets can be treated in such a way that a high quality of life is achieved following diagnosis. In this respect, it is similar to treating heart or kidney disease, chronic diseases that also can be fatal. Remember that one of the most important factors influencing a pet's quality of life and remission time is the interest and dedication of the owner and the veterinary care team.

## Response to Cancer Treatment

When trying to decide whether to continue treatment, or knowing whether treatment is successful, objective criteria are helpful. Evaluating response to treatment can often be done by physical examination but may require laboratory evaluations or imaging, as described in Chapter 4. The standardized criteria for treatment response are summarized in Table 5.1.

### Describing the Outlook with Statistics

The next section defines some terms that are often used when describing the outlook (prognosis) for a patient with cancer. These are statistical terms, and provide a guide as to how the population of animals with the same cancer type will respond to treatment; such numbers can never tell you how an individual patient will respond to therapy and how long it will survive.

**Table 5.1.** Definitions of objective tumor remissions and responses following anticancer therapy

| Tumor Response | Criteria |
| --- | --- |
| Complete (CR)* | Disappearance of all evidence of cancer in all sites for a defined period of time (e.g., one inter-treatment interval of 3 weeks). |
| Partial (PR)* | Decrease in size of all tumors by 50% or greater as measured by the sum of the products of two diameters for each tumor. These diameters should be the largest tumor diameter and the diameter perpendicular to it. There should be sustained decrease in tumor size, as defined for CR, and no new tumors should arise. |
| Stable disease (SD) | Decrease of <50% or an increase of <25% in the sum of the products of the diameters as measured for PR. |
| Progressive disease (PD) | Increase of 25% or more in the sum of the products of tumor diameters *or* the appearance of a new tumor. |

*CR + PR = Objective or Overall Response Rate.

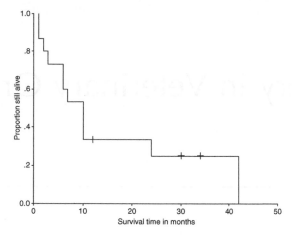

**Figure 5.1.** This Kaplan-Meier survival curve shows the progression over time of a group of dogs (see text for details). The steps represent death of a patient, and the proportion surviving can be estimated. Dogs still alive in the group are included as cross marks.

## Kaplan-Meier Survival Curve

Kaplan-Meier survival curves are one of the most common types of statistical presentations for data in oncology. These curves start with all (100%) of the animals alive (or in remission) and over time, as a patient dies (or comes out of remission), the curve tracks him/her by reducing the percentage (see Figure 5.1). The result is a series of steps.

From this curve you can calculate the median, mean, and survival rates at any time point (usually 1 year and 2 years after treatment starts). There are more examples of such curves in Section 7.

**Mean** is the average survival time of all the patients in the population being studied.

**Median** is the middle value for the survival times of the population.

An example would be a treatment for 15 dogs with stage 3, T-cell lymphoma where the survival time is measured. The survival times in months for these dogs are: 1, 1, 2, 3, 6, 6, 7, 10, 10, 10, 12, 24, 30, 34, 42. Three of these dogs are still alive at 12, 30, and 34 months. The Kaplan-Meier survival curve is seen in Figure 5.1; the cross marks show dogs still alive. For this population the median survival would be 10 months, but the mean would be 13.2 months. The 1-year survival rate would be 33.3% and the 2-year survival rate would be 26.7%. When talking to the owner of a dog with a similar disease, at a similar clinical stage (dogs with stage 3, T-cell lymphoma), you could say that there is a 50% chance that his or her pet would live 10 months or longer, and there is a 1-in-3 chance it would live more than 1 year. That actual patient may live 1 month, or it may live more than 3 years, but the *usual* survival numbers are the best information we are able to provide.

# Surgery in Veterinary Oncology

Surgery is still the modality most likely to cure an animal of cancer if the tumor is localized (not metastasized and not invading into sensitive structures). However, it is not only with curative intent that surgery is applied to pets with cancer. Biopsy, debulking, and palliation are achieved through surgery, and each needs to be carefully performed so as to minimize the impact on the patient's quality of life while still achieving the appropriate goal.

Although veterinary technicians may not perform surgery themselves, an understanding of the principles of surgery can allow them to become effective members of the oncology surgery team. Careful preparation of the patient, as well as anticipation of complications can be as important as the surgery itself in leading to a good outcome for the patient.

## Noncurative Intent Surgery

### Biopsy

When preparing a patient for biopsy it is important to clip and prepare the biopsy site, remembering that anywhere that has been cut by the biopsy instrument (biopsy needle tracts and biopsy incisions) will need to be removed when the definitive surgical procedure is performed.

After biopsy, the formation of a hematoma or a seroma might spread cancer cells as it dissects between fascial planes, which would lead to a more extensive and possibly complicated definitive surgery. The veterinary nurse should be proactive in identifying swelling after biopsy and in the careful use of dressings and bandages to reduce such complications. Remember that a drain placed to allow fluid drainage will need to be excised with its tract at the definitive surgery, as mentioned for biopsy tracts above; it may be better to avoid its use if possible.

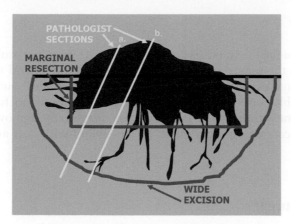

**Figure 6.1.** A schematic of an invasive tumor (such as a mast cell tumor or soft tissue sarcoma) that is sending tendrils into the surrounding tissue. With a marginal excision (pink line) the tumor will not be completely excised and will recur. With wide excision (green line), margins may be complete, but it is apparent how examination of two different parallel sections (yellow) by the pathologist would result in a different perception of the completeness of excision. If the pathologist sections at level (a), the result will reflect complete excision, whereas if the pathologist sections at level (b), the result will reflect incomplete excision.

As mentioned in Chapter 3, tissues obtained at biopsy should be carefully handled and prepared to allow evaluation of the tissue by different procedures, such as cytology and immunohistochemistry. The biopsy specimen should be handled with extreme care to prevent crushing, artifact, or alteration of the orientation of the tissue specimen. Specimens should be placed in enough preservative to allow complete fixation (a good rule is 1 part tissue to 10 parts formalin). Using inked margins or sutures may give the pathologist information regarding orientation of biopsy tissue within the body.

When the intent of surgery is to remove a large portion of the tumor, or indeed to try to cure the patient, it is important to remember that a margin (or *cuff* or *zone*) of normal tissue will also need to be removed to ensure that the tumor and its "tentacles" (Figure 6.1) will be removed. The veterinary technician/nurse should discuss this with the surgeon prior to clipping and preparing the site because the aim of the surgery and the type of tumor may mean that the amount of preparation could vary.

## Intracapsular Surgery

Also known as *debulking* or *cytoreduction*, intracapsular surgery will never lead to a cure for a cancer, but it can have a role in preserving surrounding normal tissues and structures that, if damaged, could negatively affect the patient's quality of life. Debulking will often leave behind visible tissue at the site, but it can provide palliation when a tumor is causing obstruction (say to the urethra, upper respiratory tract, or gastrointestinal tract) or pain (retrobulbar tumors or spinal tumors). Debulking surgeries require adjunctive therapy if the patient is to be cured or have a long-term remission. An example would be a dog with a mast cell tumor of the foot where limb amputation is not possible. Debulking of the tumor, followed by radiation teletherapy could be considered to have a high probability of long-term control (see Figure 6.2).

## Marginal Surgery

By this surgical technique the tumor is removed along the pseudocapsule. The pseudocapsule is formed when the tumor expands, compressing the peripheral tumor cells against the surrounding normal tissue. Grossly, the tumor appears to "shell out," but microscopic compressed (but viable) tumor cells remain and will regrow if no further treatment is performed. Again, radiotherapy is indicated for marginally removed tumors where metastasis has not occurred, and cure is still a possibility with that addition (see Figure 6.3).

# Curative Intent Surgery

When preparing a patient for curative intent surgery it is important to clip and prepare the surgery site to include any biopsy needle tracts and incisions, as well as drain holes and tracts that will need to be removed, because these could be a source of future recurrence. In addition, preparation of sites for skin mobilization or grafting should be considered. Ideally, lymph nodes should be removed at surgery and examined histologically for any evidence or tumor metastases. Removal of nodes is not known to improve outcome, but knowledge of node status can direct adjuvant therapy and influence prognosis. During surgical clipping and preparation it is important to identify any lymph nodes that the surgeon may want to biopsy. Node biopsy and skin grafting may also be considerations when positioning the patient for surgery.

## Wide (Excisional) Surgery

Excisional surgery removes a cuff of normal tissue along with the tumor contained within. Ideally, the tumor is removed en bloc, and the lateral or deep margins of the tumor are never exposed. If the margin is wide enough, a cure is possible (see Figure 6.1). However, often what appears to be a wide surgery to the cancer care team may still not be adequate. The nurse can assist in placing ink or sutures at the areas the surgeon feels least confident about so that the pathologist can specifically section and examine those sites.

Most investigators feel a clear histologic margin of 5–10 mm (depending on the tumor type) is adequate. It is important to remember that to achieve this, wider surgical margins of macroscopically normal-appearing tissue need to be removed (Figure 6.4). The published reports requiring 2–3 cm margins are clinical margins, not histologic. However, the pathology report should always be interpreted in light of the clinical impression of the surgery. If the surgeon's feeling is that the margins were not achieved, the best option is a second, "scar revision" surgery to remove margins around the remaining scar. This is true if the histopathologist does not find tumor cells at the margins, because pathologists are limited in the amount of tissue they can examine (at sections of 4 micrometers thick); this is why inking the margins at areas of concern is helpful. Thus, if the surgeon feels confident but the pathologist find tumor cells at the margin, the pathology report should take precedence; if the surgeon feels it is unlikely the excision was complete but the pathology report does not find tumor cells at the margins, the surgeon's impression should take precedence. On the other hand, if the deep margin includes underlying fascia or muscle

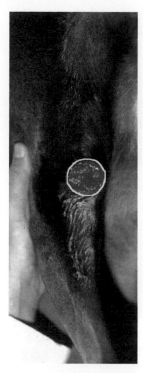 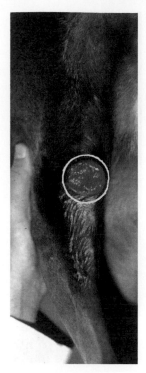

**Figure 6.2.** The yellow line denotes the approximate surgery for a debulking surgery. This surgery will not be curative.

**Figure 6.3.** The yellow line denotes the approximate surgery for a marginal surgery. This surgery will not be curative.

that has not been penetrated, these may act as a barrier to tumor invasion, particularly early on.

## Radical Excisional Surgery

Radical surgery removes a complete compartment organ or structure to achieve complete margins. The most commonly seen example is a limb amputation that could cure a mast cell tumor or a low-grade soft tissue sarcoma and be palliative for pain from a bone cancer such as osteosarcoma (Figure 6.5).

Such aggressive surgical procedures may be viewed as "mutilating" by some owners as they project their interpretation of well-being onto their pets (anthropomorphism). It is important to remember that animals often have a great quality of life with little regard for the cosmetic changes such surgeries cause.

### Amputation

Limb amputation is probably the most commonly performed of such surgeries. Although most pet owners initially do not like the idea of amputation, dogs (and particularly cats) respond to the surgery extremely well. In two studies in the U.S. and in Europe, dogs learned to walk well on three legs within a month, which exceeded most clients' expectations. All clients were happy with their decision to amputate. Pets are able to function

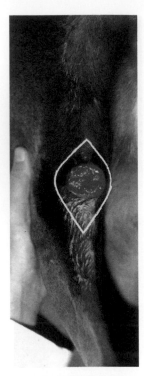

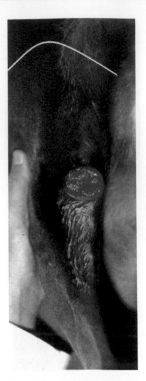

**Figure 6.4.** The yellow line denotes the approximate surgery for a wide surgery. This surgery could be curative for many tumors.

**Figure 6.5.** The yellow line denotes the approximate surgery for an amputation surgery. This surgery is very likely to be curative for any nonmetastatic soft tissue tumors at this location.

almost normally on three legs: they can go on long walks, play with family members and other pets, swim, and go up and down stairs. Most pet owners are pleasantly surprised to see how well their pets adjust to the surgery. The pain associated with the procedure is minimal, and most pets are up and around the next day. Because cats and dogs have no concept of their appearance, amputation is not associated with emotional or psychological difficulties for them.

For light, fit animals, amputation is extremely well-tolerated. (see Figures 6.6–6.9) Even very heavy dogs—if they are fit, not obese, and without significant orthopedic problems—can tolerate the procedure well. Our website has some photos and a video of dogs (including a mastiff-cross) that have undergone amputation (www.vetoncologyconsults.com/deciding_about_amputation), which may be helpful for some owners. (Another valuable website for owners of amputee dogs is www.tripawds.com.) You should always look at any website yourself before passing the address on to your clients. Finally the book *Without Regret: A Handbook for Owners of Canine Amputees*, by Susan Neal, remains an excellent resource.

### Maxillectomy and Mandibulectomy

Although most pet owners are understandably initially reluctant to have an aggressive facial surgery such as maxillectomy done for their pet, most who do are satisfied after the procedure, from both cosmetic and functional standpoints. It is important to remember

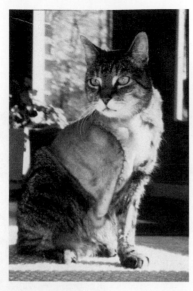

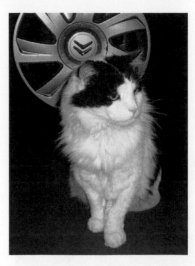

**Figure 6.7.** This cat had a hindlimb amputation some months prior and has returned to close-to-normal activity levels.

**Figure 6.6.** A cat just a few days after amputation. Pain relief following such a surgery is mandatory, but patients rapidly adapt. Cosmetically and mentally this is the worst period for their owners, but as the hair regrows concerns subside.

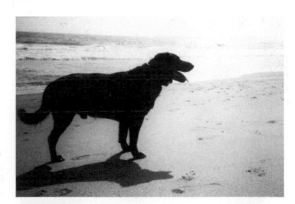

**Figure 6.8.** Dogs with three legs are able to function at a high level as pets, and participate in most normal activities. (Courtesy of Dr. Kenneth M. Rassnick)

that for pets with most oral tumors, the impact on quality of life caused by the local tumor is the most life-threatening problem; complete resection is the best way to alleviate the quality-of-life problems. In a telephone survey of caregivers for dogs with oral tumors, including some treated with partial maxillectomy, satisfaction with the surgical procedure was assessed. Overall, 85% of owners were pleased with their decision to treat their dogs, and the longer the dog had lived, the more likely the caregiver was to be satisfied. Although difficulty in eating was noted for 64% of dogs after maxillectomy, pain was felt to be less after surgery for most animals than before surgery. All clients found the cosmetic appearances of their dogs acceptable after facial hair regrew (Figure 6.10). The quality of the pets' lives was perceived by the owners to be most improved after rostral mandibulectomy (100%) and least improved after partial mandibulectomy. Similar good reports came from owners of dogs in another study.

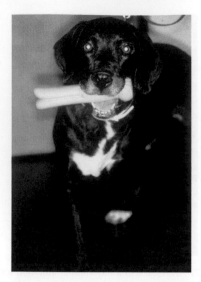

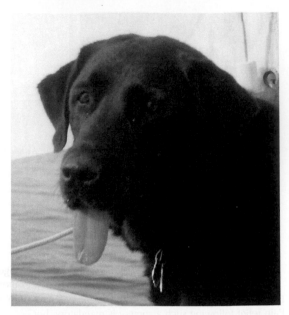

**Figure 6.9.**   Dogs remain positive after amputation and are not affected by negative body image. (Courtesy of Dr. John Berg)

**Figure 6.10.**   Mandibulectomy is an aggressive surgery, but can be curative for many otherwise fatal oral tumors. Under hot conditions, tongue "lagging" may be an obvious change (as in this yachting dog), but it is rarely a problem.

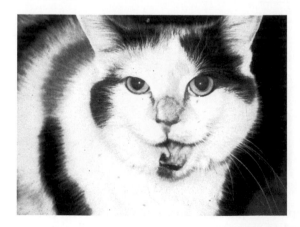

**Figure 6.11.**   Cats take longer to adapt to mandibulectomy, and continued nursing and encouragement is needed for many patients. It is still a rewarding surgery and curative for cats with many oral tumors.

A retrospective report of cats treated with mandibulectomy for oral neoplasia (all types) showed that most (~75%) cats were dysphagic or inappetent immediately postoperatively, and 12% never regained the ability to eat. Despite these findings, most (>80%) of the owners were satisfied with the outcome (Figure 6.11).

## Nosectomy

A surgery that is often used to resect a nasal plane squamous cell carcinoma in cats is a "nosectomy." This aggressive procedure is usually curative, and while the immediate postoperative period is sometimes challenging, cats recover well. Our personal pet under-

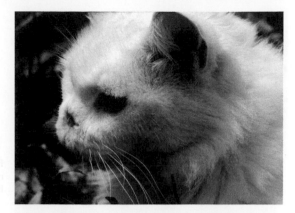

**Figure 6.12.** Nosectomy is cosmetically challenging for the owner, but once the patient's hair regrows, the normal quality of life such patients experience means that owners readily accept the physical changes.

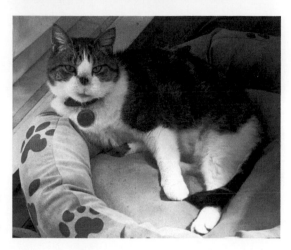

**Figure 6.13.** Cosmetic changes do not affect a cat's quality of life.

went this surgery, and lived another 6 years of excellent quality life, similar to the good outcomes seen in other patients (Figures 6.12 and 6.13).

### Brain Surgery

Cats treated for meningioma can have rapid recovery from surgery, and more than half the cats live more than 2 years. This would be considered by most owners to be a very aggressive surgery, but the quality of life for cats after surgery is excellent (Figures 6.14 and 6.15).

## Changing Instrument Packs

Because the instruments used in the resection of the cancer are potentially contaminated by tumor cells, these have the potential to be seeded into the skin and subcutis as the excision is closed. This has been seen for many cancer types but is most common with bladder transitional cell carcinomas. The oncology nurse should ensure that a clean pair of gloves and a second "closure" sterile instrument pack is available following removal of the cancer.

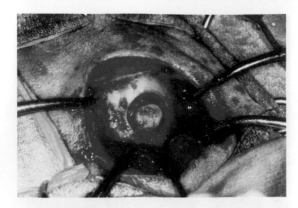

**Figure 6.14.** A meningioma is removed with resection of the overlying skull in this cat that had been seizuring. (Courtesy of Dr. Karl Kraus)

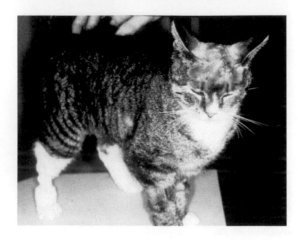

**Figure 6.15.** The same cat as seen in Figure 6.14, a day after surgery; the cat is bright and sociable. (Courtesy of Dr. John Berg)

## Further Reading

Aiken SW. 2003. Principles of surgery for the cancer patient. *Clin Tech Small Anim Pract* 18:75–81.

Carberry CA, Harvey HJ. 1987. Owner satisfaction with limb amputation in dogs and cats. *J Am Anim Hosp Assoc* 23:227–232.

Fox LE, et al. 1997. Owner satisfaction with partial mandibulectomy or maxillectomy for treatment of oral tumors in 27 dogs. *JAAHA* 33:25–31.

Kessler M. 2003. Mandibulectomy and maxillectomy for treatment of bone invasive oral neoplasia in the dog—a retrospective analysis in 31 patients. *Kleinterpraxis* 48:289–300.

Kirpensteijn J, et al. 1999. Adaptation of dogs to the amputation of a limb and their owner's satisfaction with the procedure. *Vet Rec* 144:115–118.

Northrup NC, et al. 2006. Outcomes of cats with oral tumors treated with mandibulectomy: 42 cases. *JAAHA* 42:350–360.

Ogilvie GK, Moore AS. 2006. Surgical oncology: Properties, uses and patient management, In: Ogilvie GK, Moore AS, *Managing the Canine Cancer Patient: A Practical Guide to Compassionate Care.* Yardley, PA, Veterinary Learning Systems, 174–178.

Szentimrey D. 1998. Principles of reconstructive surgery for the tumor patient. *Clin Tech Small Anim Pract* 13:70–76.

# Radiation Therapy 7

Radiation therapy (or radiotherapy) is effective for controlling a wide range of tumors in pets. Radiation therapy can be used alone or in combination with other cancer therapies, including surgery and chemotherapy. Radiation therapy is readily available to large segments of the veterinary profession through referral centers in the U.S. and in some locations in Europe and Australia.

Dividing cells are most sensitive to the effects of radiation. Tumor cells are controlled in three ways: cells damaged by ionizing radiation may be killed directly, or they may later attempt to divide and then die. Some cells remain functional but do not divide. These cells may be terminally differentiated, or they may be sterile.

Oxygen is critical to clinical responsiveness of tumors to radiation therapy. Between well-oxygenated and necrotic zones in any tumor are hypoxic cells and these are resistant to radiotherapy. Larger tumors are more likely to have abnormal blood supply and therefore more hypoxic cells; for this reason, radiation is most effective when treating small tumors or residual microscopic tumor tissue after surgery.

## Types of Radiation Therapy

Radiation therapy can be broadly subcategorized into teletherapy, brachytherapy, and systemic radiation therapy. With the exception of a few radiopharmaceuticals (radioiodine, samarium), radiation therapy is a local treatment, meaning that its effect is limited to the area it is directed to (in the same way that a radiograph images only the field of interest); therefore, care should be taken to ensure that the animal is staged properly to delineate the extent of the primary cancer, and that no metastases are present. Dogs with metastatic disease may not be good candidates for an intensive course of radiation therapy. The area to be irradiated should include margins similar to those that would be removed at wide excisional surgery. Consultation with an oncologist is essential to determine whether a particular patient with a malignancy is likely to benefit from radiation therapy.

## Teletherapy

The delivery of radiation therapy from a machine to the patient is called *teletherapy* or *external beam radiation therapy*. External beam radiation therapy primarily is delivered by linear accelerators, radioactive cobalt ($^{60}$Co) or cesium ($^{137}$Cs) source units, or orthovoltage radiation therapy machines. Because the source of radiation is external to the patient, teletherapy does not make the patient radioactive. Therefore, there is no period of isolation or quarantine required for patients treated with teletherapy.

When describing teletherapy, the dose of radiation absorbed is the most biologically relevant to tumor control and toxicity. The unit of measurement of radiation absorbed dose is the Gray (Gy). A course of radiation therapy is described in terms of the total dose, the number of fractions in which the total dose is delivered, and the time course over which it is delivered. For example, 60 Gy, given in 3 Gy fractions, 5 days a week, for 4 weeks. Most tumors in veterinary medicine receive a total dose of 40 to 60 Gy delivered in 9 to 20 treatments over 3 to 6 weeks.

### Orthovoltage Teletherapy

Orthovoltage machines produce radiation of an energy that has penetration limited to superficial tissues (about 4 cm), and the maximum dose is delivered to the skin. This means that deep-seated tumors will not receive an adequate dose when orthovoltage is used. In addition, tumors that are surrounding or surrounded by bone may have areas of the tumor "protected" due to absorption of radiation dose (bone blocks the radiation, just as X-rays are blocked from reaching a film). Orthovoltage, however, is valuable for treating superficial soft tissue tumors such as squamous cell carcinomas, mast cell tumors, or soft tissue sarcomas, and tumors within air-filled cavities, such as nasal tumors. Acute side effects are seen mostly in the superficial tissues where the highest dose is delivered, and because bone absorbs higher radiation doses than surrounding tissues, late side effects are more common in bone when orthovoltage, rather than megavoltage, is the source of radiation.

### Megavoltage Teletherapy

Radiation produced by megavoltage machines (cobalt-60 and linear accelerator) is not affected by tissue density, and deeper structures can be irradiated than when using an orthovoltage source. Maximum dose in tissues is not achieved until a depth of approximately 0.5 cm below the surface; therefore, megavoltage radiation can be "skin-sparing." Because megavoltage radiation is skin-sparing, irradiation of superficial tumors is achieved by placing a layer of tissue-equivalent bolus material over the tumor that allows dosage buildup so that the tumor is no longer "spared."

### Electron Beam Teletherapy

Electron beam therapy is available using certain linear accelerators. Electrons can be given different energies so the distance they travel varies, but then the energy reduces very rapidly. Lower-energy electrons are very useful for superficial tumors because deeper tissue is spared by a prompt fall in radiation dose—for example, a sarcoma on the thoracic wall of a cat where underlying lung must be spared (Figure 7.1). One disadvantage of electron beam therapy is the same as for orthovoltage; bone may shield underlying tissues.

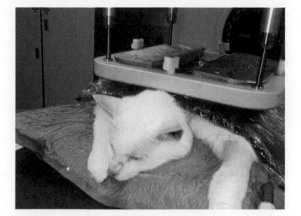

**Figure 7.1.** This cat is receiving radiotherapy for an interscapular sarcoma. The radiation must be a dose high enough to kill the tumor cells, but the underlying lung must be protected. An electron beam is being used in this patient since the depth of radiation penetration can be controlled.

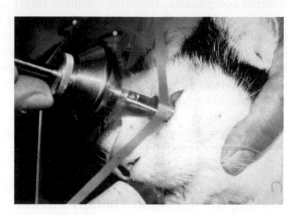

**Figure 7.2.** Strontium-90 is a radioactive source of brachytherapy that is very effective for treating shallow (<3 mm) tumors, as with this squamous cell carcinoma on the eyelid of a cat.

## Brachytherapy

Radiation therapy can be administered from implanted radiation sources ("seeds" or "straws") within or around the tumor (brachytherapy). Brachytherapy radiation has a rapid drop-off in intensity with increasing distance from the source, and it is therefore very effective for delivering extremely high doses very specifically to a local site, with normal damage usually being restricted to immediate surrounding tissues. Because the source of radiation is implanted in the patient, interstitial brachytherapy makes the patient radioactive. Therefore, there is a period of isolation or quarantine required for patients treated with interstitial brachytherapy, until their implants are removed.

Another form of brachytherapy uses an external radioactive strontium source applied to the tumor for a short period of time. This technique is most useful for shallow (<3 mm) small tumors, such as squamous cell carcinoma on a cat's eyelid (Figure 7.2), and in this situation the patient is not radioactive after treatment.

## Systemic Therapy

Radiation can be targeted to a specific tissue by use of a radionuclide with special affinity for the tumor cells. Examples in veterinary medicine include [131]I for treatment of thyroid carcinoma and $^{153}$samarium targeted to bone for treatment of bone tumors in dogs. Because the source of radiation is targeted to tissue within the patient, systemic radiotherapy makes the patient radioactive. Therefore, there is a period of isolation or quarantine required for patients treated with systemic radiotherapy, until the radioactivity is reduced to a safe level (usually less than a week).

## Treatment Goals in Radiotherapy

One of the most important decisions is whether a patient should be treated with curative or palliative intent. This influences not only the course of treatment, but also influences expectations of caregiver for their pets. Treatment with curative intent (definitive therapy) is often complicated, requiring frequent travel and multiple anesthesias. The total dose of radiation is usually higher than that required for palliation and consequently the risk of acute side effects is greater. Such treatment is likely to be prolonged and expensive; however, for many tumors the chance of long-term tumor-free survival (>3 years) is high. In contrast, palliative radiation therapy has a short-term goal, to relieve pain or symptoms of cancer when a specific site is causing a problem to the patient, but the rest of the cancer is unlikely to respond to any treatment (e.g., a painful digital metastasis from a pulmonary tumor that is not causing signs at any other site). For this reason, palliative therapy should minimize cost, inconvenience, discomfort, and risk of side effects, and should be completed in the shortest reasonable time. It is often given weekly for 3 to 4 weeks.

## Nursing the Radiation Therapy Patient

The main reason to use radiotherapy instead of, or as an adjunct to, surgery is that the marginal tissues do not have to be removed. Although cancer cells in the margins will be killed, normal marginal cells will repair and survive. This approach can enable, for example, an intracapsular excision of a soft tissue sarcoma near the orbit (rather than surgical removal of the orbit and eye), followed by radiotherapy. However, the trade-off for being able to perform a less aggressive surgery is that some side effects do occur to the normal tissues in the radiation field.

The dose (and therefore effectiveness) of radiation therapy is limited by the tolerance, and ability to repair, of normal tissues surrounding the tumor to the effects of radiation therapy. Differences in radiation response by normal tissues are determined largely by the proliferative requirements for tissue maintenance. If the proliferative requirement is high, these tissues are termed *radiosensitive* and if the proliferative requirement is low they are termed *radioresistant*. For example, liver and bone undergo little or no proliferation in steady state, but there can be a problem if there is damage that requires cellular proliferation to reconstitute normal tissue, such as a bone fracture or liver damage. Tissues that are constantly renewing, such as skin, gastrointestinal mucosa, bone marrow, glands, and reproductive tissues are considered to be radiosensitive, and these are the tissues in which the **acute effects** of radiation are most commonly seen. During radiation therapy, acutely damaged normal tissue may be repaired through recruitment of cells from un-irradiated adjacent areas.

Most normal acutely responding tissues (except bone marrow stem cells) need to accumulate a significant dose before damage is permanent, so dividing the total radiation dose into multiple **smaller dose fractions** allows repair between fractions. Increasing the size of each fraction (as with palliative radiotherapy) means the likelihood of late effects of radiation increases.

**Acute effects of radiation** are common *and should be expected* toward the end of the treatment course and for 1 to 2 weeks afterwards. Common acute side effects depending on the tumor site and surrounding field irradiated include mucositis, moist epidermal inflammation, and keratitis. The occurrence of acute effects is felt to be acceptable because healing is usually rapid and complete. In this regard, they are similar to the acute, short-term neutropenia seen after many chemotherapeutics (Figures 7.3 and 7.4).

**Late effects of radiation** are much less common than acute effects in veterinary medicine, with a prevalence of less than 5%. They are probably due to damage to vascular tissue and endothelial cells. Those tissues whose functional activity does not require cell renewal, such as muscle and nervous tissue, are more resistant to the acute side effects of radiation. However, these tissues have vascular and connective tissue stromal cells, which may be required to divide and thereby show damage that translates into late effects of radiation. Unlike acute effects, late effects of radiation occur months to years after a course of radiation therapy and are irreversible. Examples of late effects are necrosis, fibrosis, stricture formation, nonhealing ulceration, CNS damage, and blindness (Figure 7.5). The

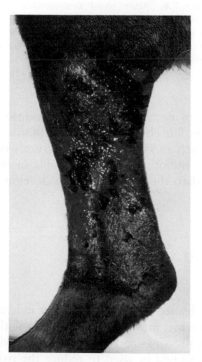

**Figure 7.3.** Acute moist dermatitis following radiation therapy to the leg of a dog with incompletely excised soft tissue sarcoma. Barrier creams, gentle cleaning and pain relief and antiinflammatory drugs should be used in such patients while healing ensues.

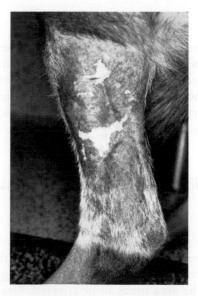

**Figure 7.4.** The same dog as seen in Figure 7.3, but 3 months later. Note the continued hair loss, but with sparse new white hair regrowth. Pigmentation is patchy, but the skin is fully healed, and the lesion is nonpainful and tumor-free.

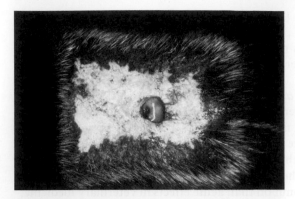

**Figure 7.5.** This dog received a very high dose of radiation and then rubbed his back (and the field) under the table causing an ulcer. The ulcer has still not healed nearly 7 months after radiation therapy, and chronic depigmentation and skin fibrosis are also evident.

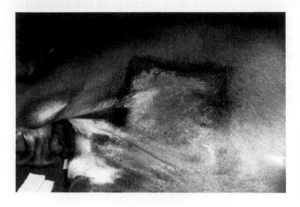

**Figure 7.6.** Acute moist desquamation in the axilla of a boxer after radiation therapy. Such areas are painful and difficult to keep dry; therefore, nursing care is very important to allow complete healing.

occurrence of late effects is dependent on the size of each radiation fraction dose and somewhat on the total dose of radiation. For example, late effects are higher with so-called hypofractionated or palliative treatment protocols such as 8 Gy per fraction given weekly than with small doses (3 Gy) given daily. Palliative radiotherapy is acceptable in many patients because their expected survival is shorter than the time it takes to develop late effects of therapy.

## Possible Tissues Injured and Possible Therapy

### Skin

Acute side effects of moist desquamation should be cleaned with saline soaks or mild soap and water if severe crusting occurs; if the area is pruritic, prevent self-mutilation with an Elizabethan collar, side bars, or bandages. Nonstick dressings/pads should be used whenever the area needs to be covered. Oral antibiotics should be used to reduce the risk of secondary infections. Other possible treatments include vitamin E and hydrogen peroxide/saline lavage, topical aloe vera gel, and hydrogels (such as Biafine) to maintain wound surface moisture (Figure 7.6).

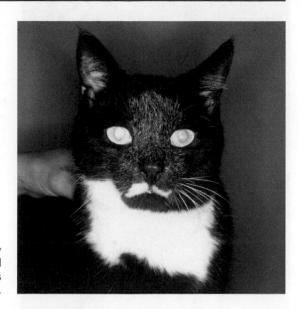

**Figure 7.7.** This cat was treated 2 years previously for nasal lymphoma, and while hair growth and healing is complete, chronic hair color changes will be permanent and limited to the radiation field.

Additional pain relief includes nonsteroidal antiinflammatories (NSAIDs) or corticosteroids in combination with tramadol, and the addition of codeine for nighttime pain when combination therapy is required. Late adverse effects commonly include changes in pigmentation (Figure 7.7), but rarely ulceration and fibrosis, which, if extensive, can be quite painful.

Debilitating late skin changes, which are extremely rare, can be repaired with reconstructive techniques using well-vascularized tissue. Figures 7.8 through 7.11 illustrate the typical course for a patient receiving teletherapy to the skin for a soft tissue sarcoma; the important point to remember is that these patients do heal, and quality of life is retained.

### Ears

Ear canals can be treated as for skin side effects, with the addition of DMSO and/or steroid-containing ear medications.

### Eyes

The eye often is in the field of radiation therapy in dogs with nasal tumors. Pain relief is as for skin acute effects. The lens of the eye is considered sensitive to relatively low doses of radiation therapy, which can result in cataract formation months to years after radiation therapy is complete. Although less common, retinal hemorrhages may result in blindness. Conjunctivitis or keratoconjunctivitis sicca may occur acutely and are painful, and it is important to monitor tear production in animals during and after therapy (Figure 7.12). For keratoconjunctivitis sicca, artificial tear preparations should be used frequently in addition to broad-spectrum topical antibiotics. It is important to confirm with fluoroscein staining that no corneal ulcers are present before prescribing steroid-containing ophthalmic ointments.

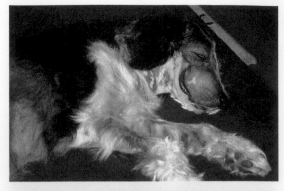

**Figure 7.8.** This dog had extensive surgery to remove a soft tissue sarcoma, but excision was still incomplete; radiation therapy was prescribed. Figures 7.9–7.11 show progression of the side effects.

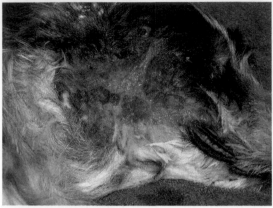

**Figure 7.9.** At the end of radiation therapy, the acute skin changes are worsening. Skin care and pain relief are mandatory at this stage, and the patient must be prevented from damaging the area.

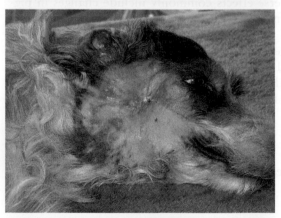

**Figure 7.10.** One week after completing radio-therapy, the acute effects are subsiding, but still present. The dog is more comfortable, but nursing is still very important to ensure complete healing.

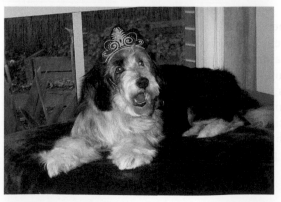

**Figure 7.11.** Four months after completing radiation therapy, this same dog feels well enough to make a dubious fashion statement.

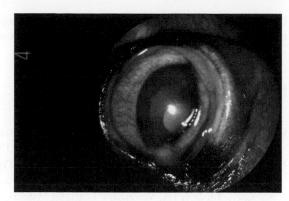

**Figure 7.12.** Acute effects of radiation to the eye are exacerbated by suppression of tear production. Controlling infection, treating pain, and replacing tears are all components of allowing full healing of the eye.

## Oral Cavity and Pharynx

Radiation-induced oral mucositis may result in anorexia and secondary debilitation. Because oral damage can be so debilitating, care should be taken to ensure that all necessary dental work is completed prior to the start of radiation therapy. Because oral and nasal damage may reduce smell and taste sensations, more palatable, warmed, aromatic foods should be offered. Placing a gastrostomy tube before initiating radiation therapy is recommended in any animal that does not have a good plane of nutrition and any time that the oral cavity is to be included in the radiation therapy field (e.g., oral melanoma in older small dogs, cats with oral SCC). Pain relief for mucositis is as for skin side effects. In addition to broad-spectrum antibiotics, consider adding metronidazole for anaerobic bacteria. During treatment, owners may want to rinse their pet's mouth out with a solution of salt and water (1 teaspoon in 1 quart of water). Cool tea solutions can be used to lavage the mouth 3 to 6 times per day, which may reduce the discomfort of the oral cavity and freshen the breath. If the patient experiences pain when swallowing, 5 to 15 ml of 2% lidocaine (xylocaine viscous solution) may be squirted into the mouths of dogs several times a day. Xerostomia may be seen as an acute effect of radiotherapy, but may less commonly become chronic, leading to dental caries. Artificial saliva preparations, such as a mixture of sorbitol sodium, carboxymethyl cellulose, and methylparaben may be beneficial in these patients.

## Colon and Rectum

Irritation to the colon and rectum can be manifested by bleeding, tenesmus, and pain. Pain relief is as for skin acute effects. A low-residue diet and a stool softener may provide relief. Steroid enemas may be beneficial in selected patients. Whenever the anus and perianal areas are injured by radiation therapy, the area should be kept clean using soap and water and dried thoroughly.

## Bone Marrow

If a significant amount of the bone marrow is included in the radiation therapy field, bone marrow damage may occur. This may be a concern when chemotherapy is also planned; in these patients myelosuppression may be enhanced. The most common scenarios would be following samarium systemic therapy for a dog with osteosarcoma or half-body radiotherapy as an adjunctive to chemotherapy for lymphoma.

## Further Reading

Flynn AK, Lurie DM. 2007. Canine acute radiation dermatitis, a survey of current management practices in North America. *Vet Compar Oncol* 5:197–207.

Moore AS, Ogilvie GK. 2006. Radiation therapy: Properties, uses and patient management, In: Ogilvie GK, Moore AS, *Managing the Canine Cancer Patient: A Practical Guide to Compassionate Care*. Yardley, PA, Veterinary Learning Systems, 148–166.

# Chemotherapy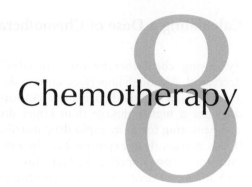

Chemotherapy is the principal modality used to treat systemic cancers such as hematologic malignancies and metastatic carcinomas or sarcomas. Many owners have preexisting ideas regarding the toxicity of chemotherapeutic drugs, and it is important to address and allay such concerns.

Although it is tempting to think of chemotherapy protocols as a "recipe" for treating cancer, in fact they should be considered as a guide. Just as every patient is an individual, each cancer is also individual, and the patient's metabolism and excretion of the drugs is individual. Complete evaluation of the cancer *and* the patient is therefore very important before administering the first dose of what are potentially very toxic drugs; for more information, see Chapters 3 and 4.

## How Does Chemotherapy Work?

In general, chemotherapy drugs are most active against cells that are actively dividing cells and in a particular phase of the cell cycle. Although most tumor cells are in an active phase of the cell cycle, only a small percentage of normal cells are actively dividing. Normal tissues can be classified as *static* (nerve, bone, striated muscle), in which the capacity for mitosis is limited; *expanding* (organs, glands), in which mitosis can be induced; and *renewing* (hematopoietic cells, mucosa, epidermis, gametes, fetal tissues), in which the proliferating proportion approaches that of tumor tissue. Toxicity from chemotherapy is most common in tissues that are renewing and is usually related to the dosage of the drug. This has implications for both the patient (toxicity and efficacy) and for the owner and veterinary staff's safety in handling the drugs during administration and follow-up care.

## Calculating a Dose of Chemotherapy

By dosing chemotherapy on a metabolic basis, the risk of toxicity to the patient is decreased. Although imperfect, current dosage recommendations are based on body surface area (BSA, m$^2$). Overall, using the BSA formula rather than body weight means that smaller dogs get a higher dosage than larger dogs (in proportion to body weight), supposedly compensating for more rapid drug distribution, metabolism, and excretion in smaller pets. If this is true, drug exposure and, by extension, efficacy and toxicity should be relatively uniform across a species. In fact, this is not so, and for veterinary use, dosage based on BSA for many drugs (e.g., doxorubicin, platinum drugs) is imperfect; cats and small dogs should be dosed at lower rates than larger dogs.

In addition, size-independent factors such as age, breed, and disease may influence drug distribution, metabolism, and excretion. Despite these limitations, veterinary oncologists use a BSA conversion table as the best practical solution, and **become familiar with the individual drugs** that require lower dosage for small pets (see Appendixes 1a and 1b).

## Dose Intensity

The concept of dose intensity is important. Dose intensity is defined as the amount of drug administered per unit time (mg/m$^2$/wk). Dose intensity can therefore be increased by increasing the dosage of a particular drug, or by shortening the time interval between drug administrations. Dose intensity should be the highest tolerated by the animal with minimal toxicity. For example, in dosing of myelosuppressive drugs, because there will be variation in individual metabolism of drugs and in the sensitivity of normal tissues, the aim should be to deliver doses that produce a *neutrophil* nadir of between 1000 and 3000/μl. There is ample evidence in both human and veterinary oncology that optimal dose intensity improves the outcome for chemotherapy.

## Chemotherapeutic Strategies in Veterinary Practice

Tumors grow most rapidly when they are small. As they grow larger, the growth rate decreases due to a decrease in the proportion of cells in active phases of the cell cycle, increased loss of cells, and cell death due to poor circulation, nutrition, and hypoxia. Larger tumors may also have a poor blood supply; thus, chemotherapy drugs may not be delivered to cancer cells at cytotoxic levels. In addition, resistance to chemotherapy can occur through spontaneous mutations in the tumor cell. The likelihood that mutation has occurred is related to the number of cell divisions that have occurred, and therefore resistance to chemotherapy is more likely in large tumors. In general, therefore, chemotherapy will be most active against small tumors, either following early detection, or following a cytoreductive ("debulking") procedure such as surgery or radiation therapy. Chemotherapy is rarely effective or curative for large bulky tumors. The exceptions to this rule would be vincristine treatment for canine transmissible venereal tumor, or combination chemotherapy for lymphoma.

## Combination Chemotherapy

Combination chemotherapy may overcome some of these problems by affecting different metabolic pathways in cells that are resistant to other drugs in the combination. Although combination chemotherapy could potentially be more toxic to normal cells, patterns of toxicity vary between drugs, and judicious scheduling of chemotherapeutic agents so that their toxicities do not overlap appears to improve tumor kill without compounding toxicity. For example, drugs that do not produce significant bone marrow suppression (such as vincristine or L-asparaginase), may be scheduled to be given 1 week after a myelosuppressive agent (doxorubicin, cyclophosphamide), or even on the same day in combination.

## Chemotherapy Drug Resistance

Although combination chemotherapy may circumvent individual drug resistance, it does not completely avoid the problem of cross-resistance to multiple unrelated chemotherapy drugs. The transmembrane pump protein P-glycoprotein is present at increased levels in some tumor cells, and both the level and prevalence increases with exposure to chemotherapy. This phenomenon of **multiple drug resistance (mdr)** occurs between anthracyclines (such as doxorubicin), vinca alkaloids (vincristine), and other drugs such as actinomycin-D, paclitaxel, and etoposide. In practical terms this means that a pet with lymphoma that is resistant to the combination of vincristine, cyclophosphamide, and prednisone (COP), may not necessarily respond to doxorubicin treatment. To reduce the risk of drug resistance occurring, it is important not to administer drugs at subtherapeutic dosages; the **highest dose intensity possible** should be delivered. It is important not to modify the planned dosages or schedule in anticipation of a toxicity that has not occurred. For example, a dog that became neutropenic after receiving doxorubicin is *not* at increased risk for myelosuppression from other chemotherapeutics such as cyclophosphamide, so their dosages should not be preemptively reduced.

## Effects of the Body on Chemotherapy Drugs (Pharmacokinetics and Pharmacodynamics)

There are four major factors that affect dosing of chemotherapeutics in dogs and cats. These factors need to be assessed for each individual patient. Particularly because many of our oncology patients are older, the effect of an aging body may significantly impact the way a dose of chemotherapy is handled, and therefore the toxic effects or the efficacy of that chemotherapy. For example:

1. *Absorption:* Orally administered cyclophosphamide may have reduced absorption from the gastrointestinal tract in an animal with malabsorption syndrome (such as GI lymphoma). This could lead to decreased efficacy of the drug.
2. *Distribution:* Drugs affected by protein binding such as vinca alkaloids, mitoxantrone, and cisplatin may be affected when an animal is hypoproteinaemic; a larger proportion of the drug may remain pharmacologically active, or may be more rapidly cleared from the body.

3.  *Excretion:* The concentration of drug in blood over time is a function of total clearance by all eliminating organs. Bile transport disruption could reduce clearance of vincristine or doxorubicin. Decreases in glomerular filtration rate may affect renally excreted drugs such as carboplatin(see box).

---

### Knowledge of Individual Variables for a Patient with Risk Factors Can Be Used to Maximize Safety and Efficacy of Chemotherapy

*Patient*: An 8-year-old neutered male Doberman pinscher diagnosed with high-grade osteosarcoma of the distal femur, 14 days after amputation. BAR, eating well, and ambulatory at home.

Preanesthetic testing revealed moderate azotemia and low urine specific gravity, but he had no clinical signs referable to renal failure. The laboratory abnormalities are stable postoperatively. How does this information affect his chemotherapy plan?

*Chemotherapy Options*: The three agents that have been shown to be most active for canine osteosarcoma are cisplatin, doxorubicin, and carboplatin. Of these, doxorubicin is contraindicated by the patient's breed because of the increased risk of cardiotoxicity in breeds predisposed to dilated cardiomyopathy. Thus, the remaining chemotherapy options are cisplatin and carboplatin, and his preexisting renal dysfunction needs to be considered:

- Cisplatin is a nephrotoxin, and any dog with underlying renal disease has enhanced sensitivity to this nephrotoxicity.
- Carboplatin is not nephrotoxic, but it is renally excreted and reduced GFR can result in increased nonrenal toxicity because of reduced clearance.

*Chemotherapy scenario 1*
The **normal** patient receiving a **standard** dose of a drug (*hypothetically* 100 units/m$^2$) will have **standard** toxicity and **standard** tumor effect.

**Clinical example:** a dog with normal renal function receiving either cisplatin or carboplatin in an appropriate administration protocol.

*Chemotherapy scenario 2*
A patient with **enhanced sensitivity** to a drug's organ-specific toxicity, receiving a **standard dose** of the drug (*hypothetically* 100 units/m$^2$) will experience **standard tumor effect** but **exaggerated toxicity**.

The same patient, receiving a **reduced dose** of the drug (i.e., 60 units/m$^2$) will experience **standard toxicity** but **reduced tumor** effect.

**Clinical example:** a dog with underlying renal disease receiving cisplatin.

If this patient receives a full dose of cisplatin, it will be effective for his cancer but will almost certainly cause severe nephrotoxicity.

If this patient receives a reduced dose of cisplatin to avoid nephrotoxicity, it will be ineffective against his cancer.

*Conclusion*: there is no safe *and* effective way to treat this dog with this drug.

---

*Chemotherapy scenario 3*

A patient with **reduced clearance** of a drug receiving a **standard dose** of the drug (hypothetically 100 units/m$^2$) will experience **enhanced tumor effect** but also **exaggerated toxicity**.

The same patient, receiving a **reduced dose** of the drug (i.e., 60 units/m$^2$) will experience **standard toxicity** and **standard tumor effect**.

**Clinical example:** a dog with subclinical renal disease receiving carboplatin.

If this patient receives a full dose of carboplatin, he will probably have a great tumor response, but he may experience severe myelosuppression, which could be life-threatening in the short term.

If this patient receives a reduced dose of carboplatin, he will experience more moderate myelosuppression and a tumor response comparable to that expected for normal dogs receiving full dose carboplatin.

*Conclusion*: by considering both drug and patient factors, it *is* possible to calculate a dose adjustment to safely *and* effectively treat this dog with this drug.

---

In fact in humans, dogs, and cats, the dose of carboplatin that most closely predicts toxicity of carboplatin is derived from measurements of creatinine clearance (as a surrogate for glomerular filtration rate). This is particularly useful in patients where there is chronic renal dysfunction.

4. *Metabolism:* Hepatic dysfunction may affect reductase metabolism of doxorubicin, thereby increasing toxicity. Cyclophosphamide requires hepatic metabolism for activation, so reduced metabolism may make efficacy (and toxicity) lower.

# Timing of Chemotherapy

**Adjuvant chemotherapy** is used following resection of a primary tumor, where the animal is at significant risk of recurrence or metastasis. The most obvious veterinary example is the effectiveness of adjuvant cisplatin, doxorubicin, or carboplatin in the treatment of canine osteosarcoma. The effectiveness of adjuvant chemotherapy is greatest at the earliest stages of growth. When a primary tumor is resected, micrometastatic foci of tumor cells have a high growth fraction and a low number of resistant cells. As a tumor grows, the growth fraction decreases, the cell cycle time increases, areas of poor vascular perfusion increase, and cellular heterogeneity increases, leading to a higher level of spontaneous drug resistance. The disadvantage of adjuvant chemotherapy is that those patients cured by surgery alone are exposed to needless risks of toxicity. For tumors such as osteosarcoma and hemangiosarcoma in dogs, and mammary tumors in cats, this percentage is small, but for animals with other tumors, the decision whether to use adjuvant chemotherapy may be less clear.

**Neoadjuvant chemotherapy** is used prior to localized treatment modalities such as surgery or radiation therapy, with the objective of reducing the size of the primary tumor and reducing the scope and side effects of other definitive treatment.

## Health and Beauty Care during Chemotherapy

During chemotherapy the pet should continue to receive heartworm preventative medication. Topical flea and tick prevention should be used rather than tablets, and dips are best avoided. Vaccination should be delayed until at least 6 months after finishing treatment. Minor dentistry or surgery can be done during periods when the pet's white blood cell and platelet counts are normal.

It usually is not a good idea to change the pet's diet too dramatically during a time when he or she is undergoing a lot of other stresses. However, we do not recommend feeding raw meat to pets that are receiving chemotherapy, because it appears to increase their risk of infection if the immune system becomes suppressed.

## Toxicity Following Chemotherapy

### Myelosuppression

*Myelosuppression* is a general term applied to the toxic effects of chemotherapy on the bone marrow. The most chemosensitive cells in the bone marrow are the proliferating hematopoietic progenitors and precursors, which are starting to commit to a particular lineage but are still immature. The more differentiated cells form a nonproliferating pool of maturing hematopoietic cells that will be unaffected by chemotherapy and will provide mature cells for 5–10 days. This means that the **nadir (or low point)** of peripheral cell counts occurs at this time. The time at which the nadir occurs also depends on the lifespan of the hematopoietic cell. Neutrophils live only hours in both dogs and cats and their nadir occurs first at 5–10 days postchemotherapy; platelets live for approximately 10 days, and their nadir occurs 1–2 weeks after chemotherapy; erythrocytes live for 120 days in the dog and 70 days in the cat, and although anemia may occur over a prolonged course of chemotherapy, it is rarely clinically significant. Like the maturing cells, hematopoietic stem cells are largely nonproliferating and so are relatively resistant to chemotherapy toxicity. However, they are stimulated to divide by the loss of proliferating precursor cells, and they rapidly replace the lost cells so that nadirs following chemotherapy rarely last more than several days. This also has implications for the interval between administrations of myelosuppressive drugs. If these drugs are given when the stem cell pool is dividing (i.e., soon after the previous administration), then severe prolonged myelosuppression due to stem cell destruction may occur. The usual interval between myelosuppressive drug administrations is every 2 to 3 weeks. Some drugs (such as lomustine and carboplatin) may have delayed or prolonged nadirs, and dosing intervals are longer for these drugs.

When administering chemotherapy, a complete blood count (CBC), including a platelet count, should be collected at the expected neutrophil nadir, usually 1 week after administration. The absolute neutrophil count (**not the percentage, or the total leukocyte count**) should be evaluated. Although many animals have a low neutrophil count without clinical signs, a count of less than 1000/μl is sufficient reason to reduce all subsequent dosages of that myelosuppressive drug. A dosage reduction of 25% is a good rule of thumb. In addition, a CBC should be evaluated immediately prior to each chemotherapy treatment. If the neutrophil count is less than 3000/μl at the time myelosuppressive chemotherapy is due, it is best to delay administration by 1 week or until the count is more than 3000/µl. A schematic for such decisions is included here as Figure 8.1; further information about patient support for pets with hematologic toxicities can be found in Chapter 13, "Hematologic Support," and Chapters 17 and 18, "Hematologic Emergencies" and "Febrile Neutropenia."

Thrombocytopenia rarely causes clinical signs, however at counts of less than 50,000/µl the risk of bleeding increases and the patient should be evaluated for petechiation, ecchymoses, or mucosal bleeding. Myelosuppressive chemotherapy should not be administered if the platelet count is less than 100,000/µl. Dogs that are thrombocytopenic should not be encouraged to perform strenuous or high-impact activities, and they are best kept at rest.

## Gastrointestinal Toxicity

Although not the most common chemotherapy side effect, gastrointestinal toxicity—particularly vomiting—is probably the one that most pet owners are afraid of when considering chemotherapy. The gastrointestinal mucosa is another site of renewing tissue, and toxicity may occur anywhere in the GI system. Clinical signs include nausea, vomiting, inappetence, anorexia, or diarrhea. The management of these will depend on the severity of signs. Severe hemorrhagic colitis following doxorubicin administration increases the risk of subsequent sepsis, due to breakdown of the protective mucosal barrier to gram-negative intestinal bacteria at a time when the animal is myelosuppressed. Antibiotics should be administered to these animals in addition to supportive and symptomatic care (see Chapter 12 and Appendix 3).

## Cardiotoxicity

In veterinary oncology, cardiotoxicity is only clinically a problem with doxorubicin chemotherapy. Although both cats and dogs show histologic cardiac changes, dogs are more sensitive to clinical cardiac damage than cats are. In dogs, cardiotoxicity is a chronic toxicity related to the lifetime cumulative dose of doxorubicin rather than the amount of each individual dosage. The damage is permanent and progressive. The end result resembles dilated cardiomyopathy, and may progress to congestive heart failure. There is no specific treatment other than palliation for heart failure, so prevention is vital. Although cardiotoxicity in dogs can occur at any cumulative dosage, it is most frequent above 180 mg/m$^2$ (in other words about six treatments at usual dosages), and doxorubicin should not be given above this level without echocardiographic monitoring. Breeds susceptible to dilated cardiomyopathy, particularly Dobermans, appear to be more sensitive to this toxicity, often developing cardiac dysfunction at doses much lower than 180 mg/m$^2$. Doxorubicin may be better avoided altogether in dogs of these breeds (see Table 8.1).

If chemotherapy with doxorubicin is anticipated, careful physical examination of the patient's cardiovascular system should be done, and if there is any question of abnormality, baseline cardiac ultrasonography is indicated. If ultrasonography shows any evidence at all of ventricular dilation or reduced shortening fraction, doxorubicin is contraindicated. In dogs with normal cardiac contractility but with preexisting valvular disease, we would **still be concerned** that the risk of worsening cardiac function is high if doxorubicin is administered. In such dogs we recommend using an effective alternative, if one exists.

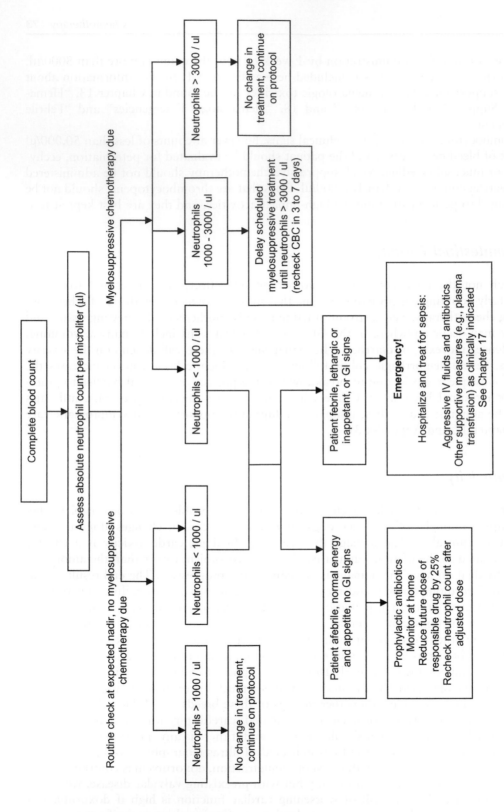

**Figure 8.1.** An algorithm for interpreting the hemogram from a dog or cat receiving chemotherapy.

**Table 8.1.** Dog breeds considered to be predisposed to cardiomyopathy and at increased risk for chronic cardiotoxicity from doxorubicin

Doberman pinscher

Boxer

Irish wolfhound

Great Dane

Cocker spaniel

Dalmatian

Newfoundland retriever (Europe)

Airedale terrier (Europe)

English Cocker spaniel (Europe)

## Urologic Toxicity

See also Chapter 22. **Nephrotoxicity** is the primary dose-limiting toxicity of cisplatin and depends on both the individual and cumulative dosage. Cisplatin should not be administered to dogs with preexisting renal disease, and it should be used with caution in dogs with urinary tract tumors. It is important to check the serum creatinine level before each cisplatin treatment. Cisplatin **should not be administered to dogs** if the serum creatinine is above the normal range and **should never be administered to cats** under any circumstances (it causes fatal pulmonary edema in cats). In addition, cisplatin should always be delivered to dogs with appropriate saline diuresis.

Doxorubicin has been associated with a cumulative nephrotoxicity in cats and should not be administered to cats with preexisting renal disease.

**Urothelial toxicity** (sterile hemorrhagic cystitis) is associated with cyclophosphamide and ifosfamide administration. Although this toxicity is uncommon following cyclophosphamide administration in animals, it will occur predictably after ifosfamide treatment in humans (and presumably pets) unless the urothelial protectant, mesna, is given concurrently. When chemical cystitis occurs following cyclophosphamide or ifosfamide treatment in pets, clinical signs of stranguria, dysuria, and hematuria can be severe and prolonged over many weeks and will be worsened by continued drug administration. This toxicity should be distinguished from infectious cystitis by bacterial culture; however, even if bacteria are isolated and signs resolve with antibiotic administration, the drug should not be administered again because infectious cystitis could have been secondary to the toxicity.

## Immune-Mediated Toxicity

See also Chapter 20. **Hypersensitivity reactions** may occur during doxorubicin administration due to histamine release. This effect occurs only with rapid administration, and it is not a problem if the drug is given as a **slow infusion** over 15 to 20 minutes. A similar, but more severe, reaction occurs following administration of etoposide and paclitaxel due to the carrier solutions in these formulations (as opposed to the drugs themselves). Both carriers cause massive histamine release, the effects of which are only partly prevented by pretreatment with antihistamines and corticosteroids.

True **anaphylaxis** may occur following L-asparaginase administration, particularly by the intravenous or the intraperitoneal route. This toxicity occurs very rarely if L-asparaginase is administered intramuscularly or subcutaneously. Attachment of polyethylene glycol (PEG) conjugates to the L-asparaginase is another approach to abrogate the immune response and extends its half-life while preserving efficacy. If anaphylaxis occurs, treatment with corticosteroids and antihistamines plus any other necessary supportive measures should be instituted immediately. The patient should never receive any further L-asparaginase.

## Hair and Coat Changes

Most breeds of dog, and all cats, have fur that is intermittently growing, rather than hair that is continually growing. Usually dogs and cats will not lose their fur, but clipped areas may be slow to grow in, and breeds that have hair that needs regular trimming (such as poodles and many terriers) may have some thinning; breeds with feathers (golden retrievers, etc.) may lose these temporarily. We have seen complete (temporary) hair loss in only one patient in over 25 years (Figure 8.2).

Cats may lose their whiskers and occasionally have a change in hair coat color. Any lost hair will grow back within a few months after chemotherapy is finished, although rarely there may be a permanent color or texture change (Figures 8.3–8.5).

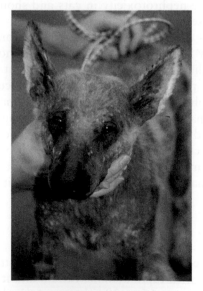

**Figure 8.2.** Complete hair loss, as seen in this schnauzer after paclitaxel, is exceedingly rare.

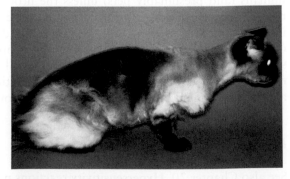

**Figure 8.3.** Fur is little affected by chemotherapy, but the longer, continually growing hair and whiskers can be lost during chemotherapy, as in this young Himalayan cat with lymphoma.

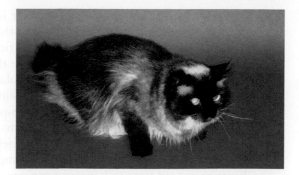

**Figure 8.4.** The same cat as in Figure 8.3, 6 months after stopping chemotherapy. This cat lived another 8 years.

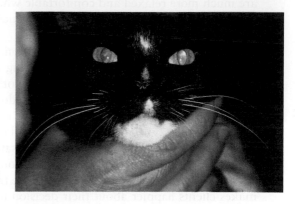

**Figure 8.5.** Whiskers in this cat are regrowing after stopping chemotherapy.

## Practical Chemotherapy

Appendix 6 contains information about availability, storage, and administration of chemotherapy drugs commonly used in veterinary practice.

### General Chemotherapy Tips

Owners should be instructed in the use of a rectal thermometer and take the pet's temperature twice a day in the period around the neutrophil nadir. A fever or any other sign of sepsis should be treated as an emergency with prompt initiation of systemic support using intravenous fluids and broad-spectrum antibiotics.

If you need a complete blood count before giving a myelosuppressive agent (to make sure the neutrophil count is above 3000/μl) and it needs to be sent to an outside laboratory, consider collecting it the day before and then arranging the chemotherapy appointment for a time when you know the results will be available.

Attention to detail is critically important in chemotherapy, from weighing patients carefully at each visit to calculate the correct dose for that day; to listening carefully to owners' comments about how the pet has been feeling; to choosing the correct drug and calculating the dose correctly; to careful administration to avoid extravasation and hypersensitivity reaction; to prescribing and dispensing at-home medications correctly. Therefore, it is very important to focus completely on the task.

1. It is necessary to clear your mind of other issues that may be happening outside of work, elsewhere in the practice, or with other patients.
2. It is very important to be able to take your time. Chemotherapy appointments should be booked with sufficient time to provide the appropriate attention without being rushed. It is important that the team calculating, preparing, and administering chemotherapy not be interrupted or hurried. Simply put, overbooking causes errors; and with chemotherapy, errors can be fatal. "Squeezing in" just one more patient seems harmless but in reality it benefits no one to schedule a complex procedure such as chemotherapy when there really isn't sufficient time available to perform it correctly.
3. Having adequate time available is also important for client and patient comfort. Clients may need time to have any concerns and questions fully addressed. Patients are much more relaxed and comfortable when the staff is not in a hurry, and as any technician knows, a relaxed patient is much easier to work with than one that is nervous.
4. Check and double-check each calculation. Having each calculation checked by another team member before administering drugs is good practice.
5. Gentle but firm restraint is critical in chemotherapy administration. Remember, these are patients you will be doing this procedure with repeatedly so you definitely do not want them to develop an aversion to the treatment room, or to you! However it is very important that the patient be well restrained during catheter placement and chemotherapy injection to avoid extravasation injury. Maintaining a fun, friendly demeanor with patients and being generous with treats before, during, and after chemotherapy helps patients remember the treatment area as a happy place. Nothing makes clients happier about their decision to pursue chemotherapy than when they see their pet is happy and eager to enter the treatment area (Figures 8.6 and 8.7).

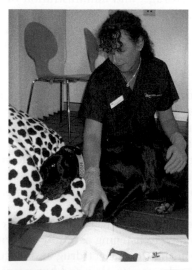

**Figure 8.6.** We find most patients are more relaxed receiving chemotherapy on the floor and with pillows for comfort and gentle restraint in lateral recumbency.

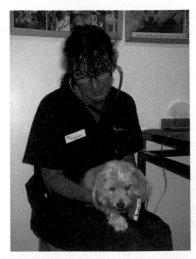

**Figure 8.7.** Some patients are best held in the nurse's lap while examined for cardinal signs, and even for chemotherapy. If this is chosen, a plastic-backed, absorbent sheet should be placed to protect the holder from inadvertent spills.

6.  Allowing clients to be with the patient during chemotherapy is very helpful for most patients. The PhaSeal system (see more to follow) makes this much more feasible by increasing the safety of the administration procedure. A few patients are better behaved when their owners are not present, but most are more secure, happier, and more cooperative when their owners are nearby. Many of our clients comment that this allows them to see that the chemotherapy process is not nearly as bad as what they had envisioned. **One exception: women who are or may be pregnant should never be allowed to stay in the room while chemotherapy is being prepared or administered, even with the best precautions in place.**

7.  Making sure that patients are physically comfortable for chemotherapy will allow them to lie still during administration. Many patients, including small dogs and cats, are more at ease being held on the floor rather than on a table. Any inconvenience to the staff in sitting on the floor is more than made up for by a more cooperative patient. Also, providing pillows for patients, clients, and staff on the floor makes everyone more comfortable and enhances the clients' sense that the practice is caring and compassionate (Figure 8.8).

8.  Place a plastic-backed pad under the limb to be used for chemotherapy administration, and use it to assemble all the equipment needed for the treatment. This includes drugs, flush, and a pressure bandage for the venipuncture site. Extra gloves, tape, and clippers should be handy (Figure 8.9).

9.  Using the smallest possible intravenous catheter for chemotherapy has several benefits. First, it is less painful for the patient, which has its own obvious benefit, but

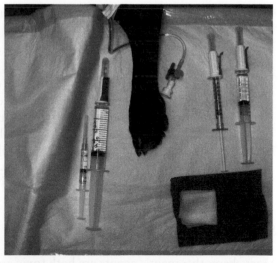

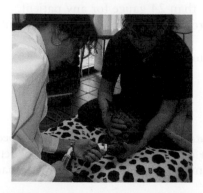

**Figure 8.8.** Even cats are more easily restrained on the floor; comfort of the pet as well as the oncology treatment staff should be considered. This cat is comfortable being prepared for chemotherapy by flushing the catheter to ensure patency.

**Figure 8.9.** Set-up for chemotherapy administration. All drugs are placed on a plastic-backed, absorbent sheet that is also placed under the patient's leg. All materials needed should be in easy reach. At the end of treatment, the sheet is rolled up and disposed of in the specially designated waste bin. When using PhaSeal, there is no risk of needle puncture, but if other systems are used, care should be taken not to remove needles, nor to recap them, but place them straight in the bin.

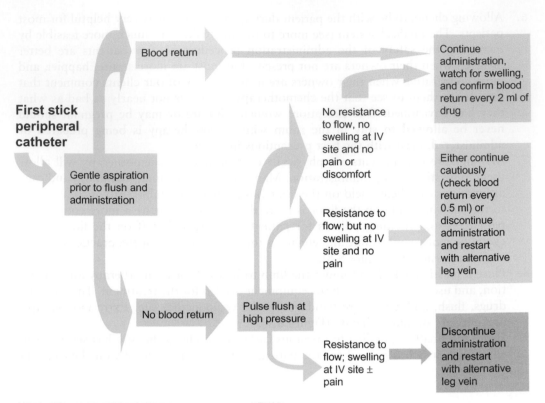

**Figure 8.10.**  When administering intravenous chemotherapy, care should be taken to ensure catheter patency, as summarized in this diagram.

also from a pragmatic point of view, they are less likely to withdraw the leg during the puncture and less likely to be anxious when they come in for the procedure next time. In addition, smaller catheters will cause less scarring, and this is especially important in chemotherapy patients because they will require repeated catheterization over time. We seldom use a catheter larger than 24 gauge for any patient.

10. For the same reason, we avoid blood sampling from the leg veins, and use the jugular vein for blood samples whenever possible.
11. Figure 8.10 provides a decision tree for giving intravenous chemotherapy.

## Safe Chemotherapy Drug Handling

Most chemotherapeutic agents are both toxic and mutagenic. Alkylating agents have been associated with the highest risks to handlers. Organ damage and increased risk of fetal loss have been reported in persons handling and administering chemotherapy with inadequate attention to personal safety.

For these reasons, precautions should be taken when handling chemotherapy drugs during any phase of preparation, administration, and disposal of drugs or waste. Ideally a vertical laminar flow biological safety cabinet should be used to prepare all chemotherapy drugs (Figure 8.11).

When administering drugs to the patient, both parenterally and orally, **latex gloves** should be worn; vinyl gloves do not offer the same protection as latex, and special chemotherapy administration gloves are thicker latex than surgical gloves (and so are preferred). Whether using a hood or not, protective eyewear, a respirator-mask and a disposable gown with closed-cuff sleeves should also be worn. All these items are usually available through distributors of chemotherapeutic agents.

Store all chemotherapy vials in zipper-lock bags in a designated cabinet or refrigerator, and if carrying syringes around your hospital with chemotherapy in them, also carry them in zipper-lock bags (Figure 8.12). During parenteral administration, **Luer-Lok syringes** decrease the risk of drug leakage or spills.

Breaking of pills should be avoided. If owners are administering drugs orally at home, gloves and waste (**zipper-lock**) bag should be provided (Figure 8.13).

All chemotherapy waste should be disposed of in a dedicated bin suitable for sharps and destined for specific commercial contaminated waste disposal. Needles should never be removed from chemotherapy syringes before disposal due to the risk of self-puncture and exposure to chemotherapy aerosols (Figure 8.14).

**Hydrophobic filters** that insert into chemotherapy drug vials will prevent aerosolization of drugs during preparation for dosing. If a filter is not used, alcohol-moistened gauze should be wrapped around the vial top and needle when the needle is withdrawn to protect from aerosolized drug.

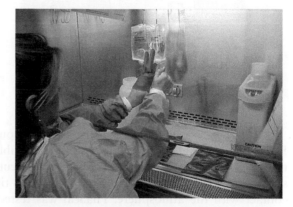

**Figure 8.11.** A vertical laminar flow hood is the ideal and safest method to reconstitute chemotherapy drugs, but it may be financially impractical for many smaller practices. Closed systems such as PhaSeal may be worth considering for staff safety.

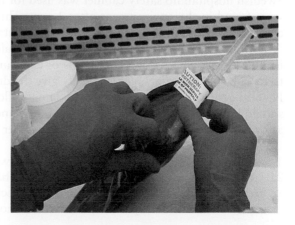

**Figure 8.12.** All syringes containing chemotherapy should be transported in zipper-locked, preferably lightproof, plastic bags. Vials of drugs should also be stored in bags in a designated refrigerator.

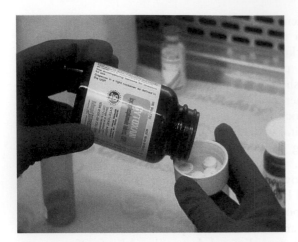

**Figure 8.13.** Oral chemotherapy should be handled with gloves, and *NEVER* split or broken.

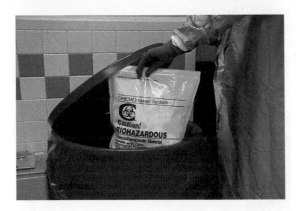

**Figure 8.14.** A designated chemotherapy waste bin should be easily accessible.

We have been using a system that is very popular in human oncology in the U.S. and Europe called **PhaSeal**. PhaSeal is a closed, double-membrane system for injectable drug transfer. The drug is transferred via a specially cut cannula and when the components are separated after transfer, the membranes act as tight seals, preventing leakage and drug contact with the atmosphere. PhaSeal was tested for 1 year in the oncology unit of a Swedish hospital: no safety cabinet was used for drug preparation, and no cytotoxic drugs were found in the environment after 1 year. This study suggests that the use of PhaSeal alone is sufficient to prevent environmental contamination (see Figures 8.8 and 8.9).

The major investment in protective effort should be at the level of preparing and administering drugs, where the higher levels of exposure to the drug occur and are more likely to be chronic (the same people usually give the drugs). We strongly suggest looking at the PhaSeal system for administration if a laminar flow hood is not available. Protective gear should be worn at all times during preparation and administration. To maximize the safety afforded by using the PhaSeal system, remember the following:

1.  **Always** handle the PhaSeal Injector by the white part of the Injector.
2.  **Always ensure that the blue injector lock is back in place *before* removing the injector from the connector or protector.** If the injector is not locked you will have an open system and increase your exposure to chemotherapy drugs.

3.  PhaSeal Injector & Connector seals are *guaranteed to remain a closed system for up to 10 needle perforations.*
4.  Wipe seals between PhaSeal product connections (i.e., Connector to Injector, Protector to Injector, Infusion Adaptor to Injector, etc.) with alcohol swab to prevent bacterial contamination.

We have found that the following methods are helpful when using PhaSeal with our patients.

### Intravenous Bolus Injections

The PhaSeal Connector is too bulky to easily attach directly to an intravenous catheter without risking dislodging the catheter. We attach the PhaSeal Connector to the delivery end of a short extension (one with a 3-way stopcock is not always necessary but can occasionally be useful). The Connector and extension are then primed with 0.9% sodium chloride, and then the patient end of the extension is attached directly to the intravenous catheter when it is placed. The injection is then given from a syringe fitted with a PhaSeal Injector that is attached to the PhaSeal Connector on the extension set. This allows a little space for the patient to adjust the position of its leg without undue risk of dislodging the catheter (see Figures 8.8 & 8.9).

### Intravenous Infusions

After attaching a PhaSeal Infusion Adaptor to the fluid bag, a standard administration set is connected to the blue end Infusion Adaptor. The injection port on the administration set is removed and replaced with a PhaSeal Connector. The line is primed with fluid from the bag. Once the intravenous catheter is placed, the patient end of the administration set line is attached directly to the catheter and fluid infusion starts. When the infusion is running well, the chemotherapy is injected into the running fluid line from a syringe fitted with a PhaSeal Injector that is attached to the PhaSeal Connector on the administration set.

## Handling Excreta from Chemotherapy Patients

The risk of chemotherapy drug exposure with handling body fluids from chemotherapy patients is a common concern for both pet owners and veterinary oncology technicians. Specific guidelines are hard to come by because no one knows what the real risks are, so people err on the conservative side. Even in the U.S. the National Institute for Occupational Health and Safety does not give specific guidelines for handling excrement from chemotherapy patients. The recommendation to avoid body fluid contact for 24 to 48 to 72 hours is therefore a "best guess" as being beyond the major excretion of metabolites from a bolus injection.

The issue of metabolites is also important because few chemotherapy drugs are excreted unchanged; most are metabolized. For example, in the 72 hours after a dose of vincristine to humans, approximately 12% of the drug is excreted in the urine (50% of which consists of metabolites), and approximately 70% is excreted in the feces (40% of which consists of metabolites). It therefore means that if a patient's companion (and dogs are gross!!) ate all the patients feces over a 72-hour period, they would ingest approximately 30% of the original dose, of which much would be destroyed in the GI tract. If they drank all the urine for that time, they would add another 6% of the dose. You can see that for a dog stepping in the urine of a patient, or an owner getting some urine on their hands one time would expose them to a miniscule amount of the original drug, and therefore probably poses a minimal risk. **The exception to this is pregnancy, and in our opinion, pregnant women should not handle any excreta from patients and should not be directly involved in giving chemotherapy at all.** For nonpregnant staff in the hospital, routine protection against excreta should reduce the risk of exposure substantially.

For drugs that are excreted in the urine (such as cyclophosphamide metabolites), the pet should be encouraged to urinate on soil where urine will drain quickly, and any urine in other areas should be handled and disposed of as chemotherapy. These precautions should be followed for approximately 48 hours following administration.

Even for a drug like cisplatin where 90% of the active drug is excreted in the urine (this is the real hazard to kennel staff), unless aerosolization occurs, the exposure is low (and also diluted and spread out over 24 to 72 hours). Therefore, it is very important to avoid aerosolizing patient urine; this means that **runs and cages must not be pressure-hosed.** Carboplatin has approximately 60% of drug excreted in the urine, so it is another concerning drug in the hospital, but much less of an issue on the grass outside.

Doxorubicin is excreted primarily as metabolites that are far less active biologically; 50% are excreted in the bile (so feces) and 10% in the urine. Again this excretion is spread out over the 24 to 72 hours.

By careful attention to details regarding personal safety, and a positive attitude toward making the environment safe and efficient, chemotherapy should be stress-free for veterinary technician/nurses.


## Further Reading

Moore AS, Frimberger AE. 2008. Anticancer drugs and protocols—Traditional. In: Kirk RW, Bonagura JD, eds, *Current Veterinary Therapy XIV. Small Animal Practice*. St. Louis, Elsevier, 305–311.

Polovich M, Whitford JM, and Olsen M. 2009. *Chemotherapy and Biotherapy Guidelines and Recommendations for Practice (Third Edition)*. Pittsburgh, Oncology Nursing Society.

Thamm DH, Vail DM. 2008. Anticancer drugs—New drugs. In: Kirk RW, Bonagura JD, eds, *Current Veterinary Therapy XIV. Small Animal Practice*. St. Louis, Elsevier, 311–314.

## Webliography

http://www.carmelpharma.com/phaseal.html (Site to learn more information about PhaSeal component systems)

# Biotherapy and Photodynamic Therapy

## Biologic Response Modifiers (BRMs)

Biologic response modification is a form of cancer therapy that seeks to control the disease, or its impact on the patient, by altering the body's responses to the cancer rather than by attacking the tumor cells directly. BRMs may

1. Stop or suppress processes that allow the growth of cancer cells.
2. Boost the cells of the immune system, such as lymphocytes and macrophages.
3. Make cancer cells more recognizable by the immune system.
4. Block or reverse processes that change a normal cell into a cancer cell.
5. Alter cancer cells to promote growth behavior like that of healthy cells.
6. Prevent cancer cells from metastasizing.

## Differentiating Agents

A treatment widely used in humans for mycosis fungoides (T-cell cutaneous lymphoma) is vitamin A analogues (retinoids), such as isotretinoin (Accutane® [Roche]). The mechanism of action of these compounds is by inducing terminal differentiation of tumor cells, and improvement has been reported in dogs. A newer synthetic retinoid, acitretin (Neotigason or Soriatane [Roche]) has also been reported to cause responses, but with less risk of hepatic toxicity than Accutane. We would suggest a 6-week trial before deciding that it is not effective; also check liver enzymes every 3 weeks for the first 6 weeks.

In a similar category is linoleic acid (safflower oil), which has been shown to cause long-term remissions, occasionally over 2 years in duration, in a small preliminary study of dogs with mycosis fungoides. The dose is 3 ml/kg body weight PO on food once daily. No clinical toxicity has been reported. Lesions that responded best were small and

in addition to TALL-104 was needed in one dog to achieve a complete remission; importantly, TALL cells are no longer available even in the U.S. (but it still shows up on owner's Internet searches).

Xenogeneic DNA vaccination with genes encoding human tyrosinase has been used to treat dogs with advanced melanoma. Median survival was >1 year, and one dog had complete regression of pulmonary metastases for nearly a year. At the end of February 2008, the USDA gave conditional licensure to this melanoma vaccine. It is only available for purchase by U.S.-based veterinary oncologists, and distribution is not currently planned to other countries for at least the next 3 years.

## Tyrosine-Kinase Inhibitors

Mutation of the proto-oncogene c-kit causes independent activation of the associated tyrosine kinase leading to development or progression of some mast cell tumors (MCTs) in dogs and cats. Two tyrosine kinase inhibitors (imatinib and masitinib) have been used to treat MCT, and both have resulted in modest activity that does not seem to be related to gene mutations. However, the recent release of Palladia (toceranib) specifically for treatment of MCTs in dogs implies that there may be a place for these agents in combination therapy for some patients.

## Photodynamic Therapy (PDT)

Photodynamic therapy (PDT) is a local cancer therapy that is based upon the interaction of a drug, called a *photosensitizer*, with light and oxygen. PDT is most useful for superficial localized tumors such as facial squamous cell carcinomas in cats. Photosensitizers are activated by light of a specific wavelength, which depends on the properties of the individual photosensitizer, and they should be inert until activated. The photosensitizer is given either systemically or topically and is allowed time to accumulate in tumor cells. Under anesthesia, light of the appropriate wavelength is then applied to the tumor (called *photoirradiation*), either by a laser or by light-emitting diode (LED) arrays, and the photosensitizer is activated and interacts with molecular oxygen ($O_2$) to generate toxic oxygen radicals.

The use of photodynamic therapy has been increasing in recent years because of technical developments in the area of light delivery systems and new photosensitizers that are cleared more quickly from the body and have fewer side effects. PDT has several advantages. It is generally relatively sparing to the normal tissues surrounding the tumor; in other words, even within the light field the normal cells are less affected by treatment than tumor cells are. Compared to radiotherapy, it requires fewer treatments, often only one, but because of the normal tissue sparing it can be repeated if needed. On the other hand it shares its major limiting factors with radiotherapy: tumor bulk and hypoxia both greatly reduce its effectiveness. Another major limiting factor for PDT has been the cost of appropriate photoirradiation equipment. However, where the equipment is available PDT can be an excellent treatment option for superficial tumors in selected patients.

# Further Reading

Bergman PJ, McKnight J, Novosad A, et al. 2003. Long-term survival of dogs with advanced malignant melanoma after DNA vaccination with xenogeneic human tyrosinase: a phase I trial. *Clin Cancer Res* 9(4):1284–1290.

Bexfield NH, et al. 2008. Photodynamic therapy of superficial nasal planum squamous cell carcinomas in cats: 55 cases. *J Vet Intern Med* Nov–Dec;22(6):1385–1389.

Elmslie RE, Glawe P, Dow SW. 2008. Metronomic therapy with cyclophosphamide and piroxicam effectively delays tumor recurrence in dogs with incompletely excised soft tissue sarcomas. *JVIM* 22:1373–1379.

Hahn KA, Oglivie G, Rusk T, et al. 2008. Masitinib is safe and effective for the treatment of canine mast cell tumors. *J Vet Intern Med* 22:1301–1309.

Isotani M, Ishida N, Tominaga M, et al. 2008. Effect of tyrosine kinase inhibition by imatinib mesylate on mast cell tumors in dogs. *J Vet Intern Med* 22:985–988.

Knapp DW, Richardson RC, Bottoms GD, et al. 1992. Phase I trial of piroxicam in 62 dogs bearing naturally occurring tumors. *Cancer Chemother Pharmacol* 29(3):214–218.

Lucroy MD, Edwards BF, Madewell BR. 2000. Veterinary photodynamic therapy. *J Am Vet Med Assoc* Jun 1;216(11):1745–1751.

Mohammed SI, Craig BA, Mutsaers AJ, et al. 2003. Effects of the cyclooxygenase inhibitor, piroxicam, in combination with chemotherapy on tumor response, apoptosis, and angiogenesis in a canine model of human invasive urinary bladder cancer. *Mol Cancer Ther* 2(2):183–188.

Schneider LA, Hinrichs R, Scharffetter-Kochanek K. 2008. Phototherapy and photochemotherapy. *Clin Dermatol* Sep–Oct;26(5):464–476.

# Complementary and Alternative Medical (CAM) Therapies

Conventional treatments are those widely accepted and practiced by the mainstream medical community.

Many owners of pets with cancer use therapies promoted as alternatives to conventional medical care, just as they choose to do for themselves. By definition, once a treatment strategy has been evaluated by clinical trials and found to be effective, it ceases to be "alternative" and enters the mainstream. For this reason, most of these remedies have little data to support or deny their efficacy. At best, many alternative modalities are harmless but unproven or have been studied and found worthless. At worst, they can be harmful either directly through toxicity or by preventing the patient from receiving potentially effective treatments.

An even greater proportion of owners of pets with cancer use "complementary" therapies at the same time as mainstream cancer treatment. Most complementary therapies are helpful adjunctive approaches that control symptoms and enhance quality of life.

Whether you agree or disagree with this approach, the veterinary oncology nurse should encourage discussion of CAM use in their patients, and should be knowledgeable about the most popular remedies and where to find reliable information for themselves and for their patients.

In humans the most widely used CAM are spiritual healing or prayer, with herbal medicines accounting for about 10% of such treatments. A recent study used a written survey of 254 pet owners to examine the use of complementary and alternative therapies in dogs and cats with cancer. In that study 76% of surveyed owners reported some use of complementary and alternative therapy; the number dropped to 65% when prayer was excluded. Nutritional supplements were the most commonly used therapy.

Veterinarians specially trained in CAM are the best source of advice for owners interested in such strategies, although unfortunately advice is often sought from people not trained in the specific area of veterinary CAM. Just as for physiotherapy (see Chapter 11), only qualified individuals should be recommended.

Traditional Chinese medicine views the body as in balance; any loss of balance between yin and yang or interrupting the flow of Qi will result in illness including cancer.

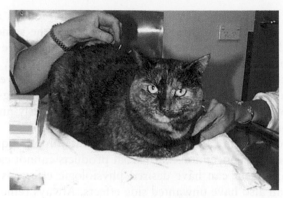

**Figure 10.1.** This cat is receiving acupuncture. As a complement to surgery, radiotherapy, or chemotherapy, acupuncture may assist in pain control and reduce nausea. (Courtesy of Dr. Pamela Short)

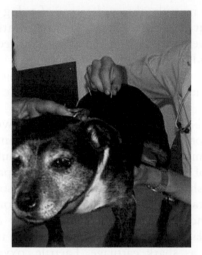

**Figure 10.2.** A dog receiving acupuncture. This procedure needs to be performed by highly trained and skilled individuals to obtain maximum benefit to the patient. (Courtesy of Dr. Pamela Short)

Examination of tongue coating or color, bodily scents, and pulse assessment may lead to a specific diagnosis that can be treated with herbal formulas and/or acupuncture. Acupuncture may also reduce nausea, vomiting, and fatigue from chemotherapy and radiotherapy, and may be a part of multimodality pain control (Figures 10.1 and 10.2).

Naturopathy relies on herbs, nutrition, and manipulation/massage, and therefore there is crossover between naturopathy and herbal medicine. Many mainstream cancer treatments have also originally come from herbal sources, such as vincristine from the periwinkle plant and paclitaxel from the yew tree.

Dietary supplements and herbal remedies rely on low doses of chemicals to have their effect. However, health regulatory bodies have not evaluated such remedies for safety and effectiveness, and few undergo any formal quality control. Some herbal remedies can interact with chemotherapy drugs, increase sensitivity of skin to radiation therapy, and interact with anesthetics. Those interactions documented in humans include feverfew, garlic, gingko, and ginger as anticoagulants, which could be a problem if NSAIDs are also administered as part of therapy. The risk of drug-herb interactions appears greatest in human patients with liver or renal disease, and we presume the same for animals. Two popular human herbal remedies for cancer in the U.S. and Europe are Essiac, a combination of burdock, sorrel, slippery elm and turkey rhubarb; and Iscador, a mistletoe extract. Neither has shown activity in human clinical trials. Mushroom-derived compounds have shown some benefit in human trials, but in the only clinical trial in dogs reported, Maitake extract had no effect when used alone to treat dogs with previously untreated lymphoma, and median time to progression was less than 1 month.

One of the major concerns in cancer treatment is maintaining the quality of life of our patients. It is a common misconception that herbal products cannot cause side effects. By definition, any substance that can have desired physiologic effects is pharmacologically active and therefore can also have unwanted side effects. Always remember that a patient receiving herbal supplements can develop toxicity from those as well as from chemotherapy. When toxicity cannot be explained by the traditional therapy, other treatments should be examined. An unwell patient should have all medications ceased (not just the mainstream treatments). We recently observed a case of a dog receiving doxorubicin and vincristine chemotherapy that developed severe and symptomatic liver damage. It was only when herbal supplements were ceased that the dog recovered. That dog was receiving five-mushroom extract, liquid herbal formula (Withania, St Mary's thistle, Marshmallow, Astragalus, Panax ginseng, tumeric), Xue Fu Zhu Yu Tang, AntiOx Excel, Protexin, and fish oil in addition to the conventional treatments. It is easy to see how this can be confusing.

Dietary antioxidants (herbal or chemical) may interfere with the efficacy of chemotherapy and radiotherapy. Both treatments cause oxidative damage as part of their cancer cell killing, so antioxidants may protect normal tissue but could also protect cancer cells from therapy. Most trials of antioxidants for both cancer prevention and with cancer treatment in humans have shown little to no benefit, and some have shown increased mortality in cancer patients taking antioxidant supplements compared to those not taking supplements. We recommend cessation of all antioxidants during chemotherapy and radiotherapy courses for 3 days before and 4 days after each treatment.

Biologic treatments such as shark cartilage, Laetrile, oxygen, and ozone therapies; insulin potentiation therapy; coffee enemas, and immunoaugmentation therapy are often supported by compelling anecdotes and testimonials, but definitive clinical trials have yet to conclusively support or deny activity. Until such time as these trials are completed, such therapies should not be recommended as a replacement for proven therapies. Common questions come from owners that find encouraging-sounding remedies on Internet searches. Our personal opinion is that these are commercialized products with no proven efficacy. The tone of the websites is very positive, and there are many testimonials, but these treatments cannot be recommended to replace mainstream treatments until controlled studies have been performed and reported.

Homeopathy describes serial dilutions to extract the vital essence of a substance, to the point where no measurable substance exists. There is no scientific data in the veterinary literature to support the efficacy of homeopathy, and it should not be offered as an alternative to standard treatment for cancer.

Nonetheless, it should be understood that owners of pets with cancer are distraught and want to pursue any and all avenues that may benefit their pet in any way. From a medical standpoint, the safest thing for the pet is to keep communication open about what the pet is receiving, and open communication is best maintained in an atmosphere that conveys understanding and support. Emphasizing to pet owners that the primary goal of conventional veterinary oncology is to maximize quality of life, and that the efficacy of possible treatments is always weighed against any quality-of-life impact, often helps to allay pet owners' fears and increase their level of trust in the team.

## Warning Bells

Pet owners should be wary when

1. The treatment claims to cure all cancers.
2. The practitioner asks them not to tell their veterinarian.
3. The treatment is claimed to have positive results with no side effects.
4. Clinical studies are claimed but cannot be provided.
5. The alternative remedy is a "secret."
6. The practitioner does not have any qualifications.
7. The practitioner attacks the mainstream medical establishment.

## Further Reading

Bjelakovic G, Nikolova D, Gluud LL, Simonetti RG, Gluud C. 2007. Mortality in randomized trials of antioxidant supplements for primary and secondary prevention: systematic review and meta-analysis. *JAMA* 297(8):842–857.

Cassileth BR, Deng G. 2004. Complementary and alternative therapies for cancer. *The Oncologist* 9(1):80–89.

Griessmayr PC, Gauthier M, Barber LG, et al. 2007. Mushroom-derived Maitake PETfraction as a single agent for treatment of lymphoma in dogs. *JVIM* 21:1409–1412.

Lana SE, Kogan LR, Crump KA, Graham JT, Robinson NG. 2006. The use of complementary and alternative therapies in dogs and cats with cancer. *J Am Anim Hosp Assoc* Sep–Oct;42(5):361–365.

Rijnberk A, Ramey DW. 2007. The end of veterinary homeopathy. *Australian Vet J* 85(120):513–516.

# Section 4

Supportive Care of Patients

# Comfort, Pain Management, and Physical Rehabilitation

*Patricia Suomala*

*Note:* For the analgesics discussed in this chapter, doses can be found in Appendix 2.

## The Multimodal Support Nursing Paradigm

The veterinary cancer patient's daily comfort level is of utmost importance to all involved in their treatment and is a key indicator of perceived quality of life for pet owners. The veterinary cancer team should inform and educate pet owners about the disease, its course of treatment, and the support available to them, and assist in assessment of quality of life. When you are communicating with owners, it is important that realistic expectations and parameters are established so that as the veterinary cancer patient enters the final stages of disease the team can provide the best possible care. This should include a multimodal approach that includes pain relief, physical rehabilitation/therapy, environmental (home) adaptive care, nutritional support, quantifying quality of life, hospice care, and bereavement support. The chapters in this section will introduce the veterinary nurse and technician to the principles and practicalities of pain relief, physical rehabilitation/therapy, nutritional/ gastrointestinal support, hematologic support, and end-of-life supportive care.

One must have some sense of how to measure and quantify well-being for each patient, and importantly owners need to have some expectations of what they feel is a quantifiable quality of life. Empower your clients with knowledge; they deserve to know the truth about all aspects of their pet's cancer care. As a veterinary nurse, you should strive to be able to assess veterinary patients for pain and comfort each time you interact with them.

Nurses have a role in all the following stages of pain management for cancer patients:

1. *Assess patient.* Pain should be assessed at the same frequency and on the same schedule as temperature, heart rate, respiration, and blood pressure.

2. *Provide nonpharmacologic comfort.* Nurses are adept at "reading" patients, particularly oncology nurses, who know their patients much better than those dealing with acute care, and they understand the emotional needs of the patients. Physical therapy (see later in this chapter) can provide comfort, and it is often used as a way of contacting patients without intrusive procedures (such as venipuncture, rectal temperature, etc.). For specific pain sites, either hot or cold compresses may provide some comfort. Providing clean dry cages, with soft padded bedding and a comfortable temperature, should never be overlooked (Figure 11.1). Restraint for any procedures should be gentle and with due consideration to the patient's history of injury and illness (Figures 11.2–11.4). For hospitalized patients, a light dimmer switch will allow for a quieter, more settled environment.

   Invasive procedures should be planned to minimize noxious stimuli (for example, coordinating blood sampling and intravenous catheter placements). One author has suggested that interventions that are invasive be balanced with positive, noninvasive interaction at a ratio of 3:1 (noninvasive:invasive); this makes intuitive sense. Such procedures are very important and, while not a substitute for analgesia, should be considered part of the multifaceted approach to pain relief and recommended to owners as a prophylactic strategy for their pets.

3. *Differentiate signs of pain from other effects.* This may take into account breed factors (huskies and malamutes may vocalize even when not painful, but when stressed or threatened) as well as anxiety levels (Figure 11.5).

4. *Request and administer appropriate analgesia.* Where possible, predict how painful a procedure will be and use prophylactic control. Include assessment of underlying factors, breed and individual factors, drug contraindications, and history.

5. *Monitor and treat adverse effects of analgesic drugs.* One study showed that in an ICU setting, only 64% of pain medications were delivered as prescribed, and nearly a quarter of patients received a decreased dose of the prescribed drug (usually opioids). This was principally done by increasing the interval (delaying administration). The reasons appear to be concern about sedation, hypotension, and hypothermia; but remember that pain has effects as well that may be worse.

6. *Communicate with clients.*

7. *Track controlled substances.*

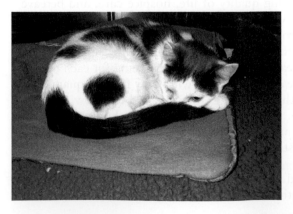

**Figure 11.1.** Soft, warm bedding is one of the most basic comfort measures and will help to reduce pain from any source.

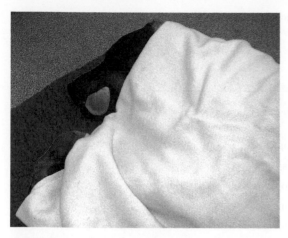

**Figure 11.2.** When recovering from anesthesia, the patient should be in an area where it is quiet, but also where it can be observed for worsening signs of pain. Again, the patient should be warm and comfortable.

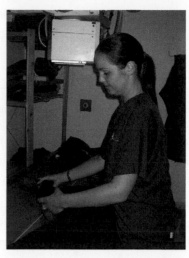

**Figure 11.3.** Gentle restraint, and judicious use of sedatives, allows for relatively pain-free procedures such as radiography.

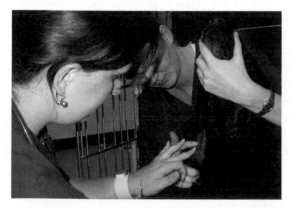

**Figure 11.4.** Gentle restraint for procedures such as blood drawing should be interspersed with noninterventional interactions (patting and feeding) to lessen anticipation of pain.

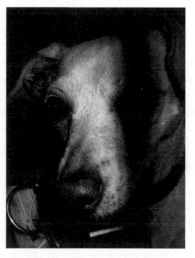

**Figure 11.5.** Nervous animals out of their normal environment may experience heightened pain that can be at least partly reduced by gentle and thoughtful nursing.

## Attitudes toward Pain in Veterinary Nursing

In a study of over 500 veterinary nurses (see Table 11.1), 58% believed that the responsibility for postoperative pain monitoring should be shared between the veterinary nurse and the veterinarian, more than 80% of the veterinary nurses agreed that a pain scale was a useful clinical tool, and 96% of them felt their knowledge and assessment of pain could

**Table 11.1.**   Percentage of 517 veterinary nurses agreeing with statements about pain (Coleman and Slingsby 2007)

|  | Agreed | Disagreed |
|---|---|---|
| A degree of pain is required to stop the animal from being too active after surgery. | 24.0 | 76.0 |
| Animals benefit from perioperative analgesic therapy. | 95.0 | 5.0 |
| Animals benefit from postoperative analgesic therapy. | 90.0 | 10.0 |
| Surgery does not usually result in sufficient pain to warrant analgesic therapy. | 1.3 | 98.7 |
| Animals recover better from anaesthesia if given analgesic therapy. | 91.9 | 8.1 |
| A pain scale to assess a patient would be/is a useful clinical tool. | 80.3 | 19.7 |
| Pain could be better assessed in animals. | 88.8 | 11.2 |

be improved. That same study showed that when veterinary nurses were asked to score pain, they scored pain higher than veterinarians for all surgical procedures. In addition, the longer a nurse was qualified the more likely he or she was to assign a higher pain score to a procedure. More than one study has shown that the pain scores given by veterinarians and by nurses for procedures involving dogs are higher than those involving cats.

One survey by a veterinary technician found that the majority of veterinarians, when asked, "How do you know an animal is in pain?" included "because my technician tells me" within the top 10 reasons on their lists. This emphasizes the importance of veterinary nurses in the process of pain management.

## Physiology of Pain

The International Association for the Study of Pain defines pain as "an unpleasant sensory and emotional experience associated with actual or potential tissue damage, or described in terms of such damage." Awareness of animal pain has been delivered to the forefront of veterinary medicine due to the support of multiple organizations within the veterinary medical community, including The American Animal Hospital Association (AAHA), The International Veterinary Academy of Pain Management (IVAPM) and The Veterinary Anesthesia and Analgesic Support Group. AAHA has made pain management part of the mandatory standards of care, as follows:

*Mandatory Standard Pain Management*:

**MA23** Pain assessment is considered part of every patient evaluation regardless of the presenting complaint.

**MA24** Appropriate pain management is provided for the anticipated level and duration of pain.

Both pet owners and the veterinary community embrace these standards.

As a veterinary nurse, you need to know how to identify the different types of pain that affect our veterinary cancer patients and methods to score and assess pain; you also must be able to communicate your assessment to the veterinarian so that the most effective analgesic provides comfort and control in the most appropriate delivery system.

Pain as defined by The International Veterinary Academy of Pain Management involves a complex interaction of physiochemical responses leading to the perception of an unpleasant sensation. Pain recognition involves transduction, transmission, modulation and perception. **Transduction** is defined as the translation of noxious stimuli processed by the peripheral receptors and is inhibited by NSAIDs, opioids, and local anesthetics. **Transmission** is the communication of noxious stimuli to the spinal cord and is reduced by local anesthetics and alpha-2 agonists. **Modulation** refers to the adjustment of noxious sensations by neurological tracts within spinal cord pathways and the brain stem and is influenced by local anesthetics, alpha-2 agonists, opioids, NSAIDs, tricyclic antidepressants (TCAs), serotonin-selective reuptake inhibitors (SSRIs), and NMDA receptor antagonists. **Perception** refers to the interpretation of noxious stimuli in the brain, resulting in sensation of pain; this is the part of pain that shows the most individual variation. Perception is inhibited by general anesthetics, opioids, and alpha-2 agonists.

Pain may be classified as **physiologic**, which refers to the body's protective mechanism to avoid tissue injury, or **pathologic**, which arises from tissue injury and inflammation or damage to a portion of the nervous system. Pathologic pain may be further separated into nociceptive (peripheral tissue injury), neuropathic (damage to peripheral nerves or spinal cord), visceral (stimulation of pain receptors in the thoracic or abdominal viscera), and somatic (injury to tissues other than viscera, such as bones, joints, muscles, and skin). Cancer pain is associated with tumor invasion and tissue damage that causes activation of pain receptors. An example is the pain caused by lysis and microfractures due to osteosarcoma in both dogs and cats. Also, cancer treatment sometimes results in pain (e.g., surgery, acute effects of radiation, and extravasation of certain chemotherapeutic drugs).

## Assessing Pain in Animals

It can be difficult to evaluate pain in animals because of the communication barrier. In human medicine there are pain scales based on numerical denominators. An example of a nonnumeric, nonverbal pain scale used in human pediatric medicine is based on facial expression. However, even this is difficult to use in veterinary medicine because while our patients do have some modulation of facial expression, it does not correlate with established parameters for human pediatrics.

Behavior and measurement of physical parameters are probably the best surrogates for the parameters we use in humans (verbal communication and facial expression). Physical parameters include heart rate, respiratory rate, and response to physical manipulation. Behavioral parameters include hiding, withdrawal from contact, aggression, and even self-mutilation.

Because of the complexity of animal pain, it is helpful to develop a standard pain form or protocol in your specific veterinary hospital so that each veterinary team member is evaluating each patient based on similar physical factors and behaviors. A semiquantitative scale for rating pain can be as simple and easily applied as "*No Pain/Mild Pain/Moderate*

**Table 11.2.**  Example of a pain score system

| Category | Sign | Score |
|---|---|---|
| Behavior | Vocalizing | 1 |
| | Shivering (if not hypothermic) | 1 |
| | Change in behavior, e.g., hiding and quiet when normally gregarious, or unusually solicitous | 1 |
| | Restless, depressed, or irritable | 1 |
| | Unusual posture, e.g., hunched | 1 |
| | Reluctant to move, soils itself | 1 |
| | Looks at, chews, or licks wound | 1 |
| | Bites at bandage | 1 |
| | Responds slowly to stroking (nonaggressive pet) | 1 |
| Socialization—for a normally nonaggressive animal | Responds slowly to gentle physical interaction, e.g., petting | 1 |
| | Does not respond to gentle physical interaction, e.g., petting | 2 |
| | Responds with fear or aggression to gentle physical interaction, e.g., petting | 3 |
| Heart rate | 11–30% increase over resting | 1 |
| | 31–50% increase over resting | 2 |
| | >50% increase over resting | 3 |

*Pain/Severe Pain.*" A more detailed example is given in Table 11.2. Regardless of the pain scale being used, it is very important to communicate the details to each staff member and ensure that evaluations are recorded in each patient's medical record.

## Multimodal Pain Management

Once the pain assessment is completed it is useful for the practice to have a standardized approach depending on the degree of pain. Table 11.3 is an example of such an approach.

An example of a real-life cancer situation where pain relief is a very important aspect of treatment is osteosarcoma in dogs (Figure 11.6). Bone pain is notoriously refractory to medical management. Amputation is the most direct method to relieve pain, and postoperative pain control is much easier than control of bone pain in patients not undergoing amputation. For owners that are not interested in amputation, or for patients in whom it is not feasible, the following options are available. As with arthritis pain, there is great individual variation in response to different drugs, so it's necessary to experiment for each individual dog:

**Table 11.3.** Example of a multimodal pain management plan

| Degree of Pain | Pharmacologic Analgesic | Nonpharmacologic Therapy |
|---|---|---|
| Mild | + Nonopioid (e.g., NSAID) | ± Physical therapy<br>± Adaptive home care<br>+ Nutritional assessment |
| Moderate | + Nonopioid (e.g., NSAID)<br>+ Tramadol<br>± Opioid | + Physical therapy<br>+ Adaptive home care<br>+ Nutritional assessment |
| Severe | + Nonopioid (e.g., NSAID)<br>+ Tramadol<br>+ Opioid<br>± Anxiolytic<br>± Palliative procedure (e.g., radiation)<br>± Other (e.g., bisphosphate) | + Physical therapy<br>+ Adaptive home care<br>+ Nutritional assessment<br>± Nutritional support<br>+ Nursing/hospice care |

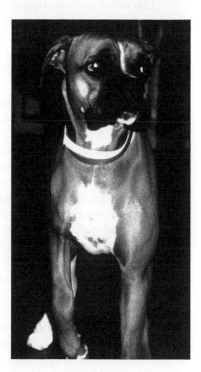

**Figure 11.6.** This young boxer has an osteosarcoma affecting the right distal radius. Although amputation is the most direct and effective method of pain control, other strategies will help improve his comfort level until surgery can be scheduled.

1. Nonsteroidal antiinflammatories can be helpful but usually do not control the pain themselves. Piroxicam, carprofen, or meloxicam can be tried, but of course they cannot be combined with each other due to an increased risk of gastrointestinal side effects. There is no single best agent for all dogs and experimenting to find the best choice for the individual dog is sometimes necessary. In one study over 75% of osteosarcoma samples showed COX-2 expression, although the staining was "strong" in only 10%

of these. For these latter dogs, the prognosis was worse for long-term survival. Piroxicam (but not other NSAIDs to date) has been shown to have some antitumor effects in tumors with strong COX-2 expression and may therefore be a consideration for therapy.

2. Corticosteroids are not usually particularly helpful, but they can be tried; however, they must not be combined with NSAIDs due to an increased risk of gastrointestinal side effects.

3. Tramadol works through complex interactions between opiate, adrenergic, and serotonin receptors. Because it is not a narcotic, it can be combined with NSAIDs and opioids to reduce the effective dosage of all drugs.

4. Narcotics can be combined with NSAIDs and tramadol. Whenever instituting a new narcotic therapy, there is a possibility that sedation will occur; this usually will pass in the first few days of treatment. We don't usually combine different narcotics with each other, especially at home.

   Codeine is often helpful, particularly for "breakthrough" pain at night, and is easy for owners to manage and adjust at home. We recommend starting at the low end of the dose range and working up, according to the patient's levels of pain and sedation.

   The other narcotic option that is certainly convenient, although less commonly successful (in our opinion) than codeine, is a fentanyl transdermal patch. It is quite safe to the dog but if there are children in the house it should be avoided because of the small but serious risk that a child might remove or find and ingest the patch. Some people find it difficult to get the patches to stay on and get frustrated with it. If a fentanyl patch is used it can take 24 hours for blood levels to rise, so dogs can be given a "loading dose" of injectable fentanyl intravenously. Note that fentanyl patches can be used in cats with a decreased surface exposure (less of the backing removed) to modify dosages.

5. A single dose of radiation therapy provides some degree of pain relief in 80% of dogs for a median duration of 4 months. It can take up to 2 weeks for pain relief to become apparent. This option can be combined with any of the medical analgesia discussed above. Some clinicians (including us) like to give 1 fraction and then "save" the further fractions for when pain recurs.

   A second radiation therapy option for osteosarcoma is samarium treatment. Samarium is a radioactive isotope that is directed to areas of increased bone turnover. The emitted radiation travels only a short distance, so it irradiates the tumor (where it accumulates) and very little surrounding tissue. Because it is taken up in small amounts by all the long bones, samarium can be myelosuppressive, at least in the short term. Thus it cannot easily be combined with myelosuppressive chemotherapy. Samarium is only available at specialized facilities.

6. Although not an analgesic, per se, for bone pain, aminobisphosphonates can be part of a multimodality approach to pain control. Aminobisphosphonates inhibit osteoclast activity and so can reduce and, in some cases, partially reverse osteolysis and the resultant pain and fracture risk. Again, it can take up to 2 weeks for pain relief to become apparent. Aminobisphosphonates are a mainstay of treatment for humans with multiple myeloma or bone metastases. These can be combined with both analgesic drugs and radiation therapy. Both alendronate and pamidronate have been anecdotally reported to be safe and effective in dogs. Pamidronate is given as an in-hospital infusion every 3 weeks; this option is fairly expensive. Alendronate is given daily at home, but it must be given after a 12-hour fast and no food can be given for 30 minutes after

the dose. Esophageal irritation can occur particularly in patients that lie down after taking the drug, so a drink of water immediately after, followed by a walk, is recommended to prevent lodging of the tablet in the esophagus.

## Pharmacologic Analgesic Therapy

In selecting pain control drugs, consider their mechanism of action, potency, duration of efficacy, effects on the central nervous system, antiinflammatory effects, toxicity, drug interactions, and cost. Analgesics when used correctly and concurrently will result in effective pain management while using lower doses of each drug. Pharmacologic methods should be used in conjunction with nonpharmacologic methods such as physical therapy, adaptive home care, and palliative therapy.

### Opioids

Opioids are the most powerful analgesics available with actions at peripheral, spinal and supraspinal levels.

There are four types of opioid receptors with multiple receptor subtypes:

1. Mu receptors produce the most profound analgesia and they can cause euphoria, respiratory depression, physical dependence, and bradycardia.
2. Kappa receptors trigger a lesser analgesic response; side effects can be sedation and dysphoria.
3. Delta receptors modulate mu receptor activity.
4. Sigma receptors provide little to no analgesia; they are responsible for many of the adverse affects associated with opioids.

Opioids may act as agonists, antagonists, partial agonists, and mixed agonist/antagonists. Simply put, as their names imply, agonists bind and stimulate receptors; antagonists bind and block or inhibit receptor activity; partial agonists bind and stimulate, but with less than full activity at certain receptor subtypes; and mixed agonists/antagonists stimulate some receptors while blocking others.

Table 11.4 lists some opioids used in veterinary medicine.

### Nonsteroidal Antiinflammatories

Nonsteroidal antiinflammatory drugs (NSAIDs) remain the core therapy for chronically painful pets. Their principal mode of action is to block prostaglandin production by

**Table 11.4.**   Common veterinary opioids

| Opioid Agonists | Opioid Agonist/Antagonists |
| --- | --- |
| Fentanyl | Buprenorphine |
| Codeine | Butorphanol(not considered effective in chronic pain) |
| Morphine | L-Methadone |

# Veterinary Physical Rehabilitation

Physical rehabilitation, or physical therapy, of the veterinary cancer patient should center on the patient's quality of life and disease process. Older cancer patients can suffer from degenerative diseases, for example, osteoarthritis; younger dogs may be top canine athletes prior to their diagnosis. A veterinarian should evaluate each individual patient fully before any physical rehabilitation begins. Unless the nurse is specifically trained in physiotherapy, it is preferable to involve a qualified physiotherapist who best understands the methods and limitations. Veterinary physical rehabilitation is often unsuccessful in animals where their underlying pain and disease state is not evaluated and treated appropriately. Because veterinary cancer patients range in age and disease pathology, one must keep in mind that the goal of rehabilitation is to provide comfort while assisting owners in letting their pet live the best quality of life possible. With that in mind, the veterinary nurse can benefit from the following brief introduction to physical therapy and contribute to creating a plan for their patients.

The American Physical Therapy Association defines physical therapy as the science of the application of biomechanics, physics, anatomy, physiology, and psychology to persons with dysfunction, injury, pain, or physical abnormalities. Veterinary physical therapy is defined by the American Veterinary Medical Association (AVMA) as the use of noninvasive techniques, excluding veterinary chiropractic, for the rehabilitation of injuries in nonhuman animals.

In the U.S., veterinary physical therapy should be performed by a licensed veterinarian; a veterinary or animal health technician licensed, certified, or registered in veterinary physical therapy or rehabilitation; or a licensed physical therapist educated in nonhuman animal anatomy and physiology.

The goal of rehabilitation is to return to predisease or preinjury function. In instances where return to normal function is limited (e.g., after amputation of a limb for osteosarcoma), the goal of rehabilitation would be to heal the affected limb site and rehabilitate the patient to strengthen the remaining limbs for function. Tissues most affected by immobilization are cartilage, muscle, ligament, tendon, and bone. The knowledge of how and in what period these tissues respond to disuse and immobilization is an important concept in physical therapy and understanding how to safely remobilize tissues after injury and immobilization is key to successful rehabilitation and quality of life. The benefits of rehabilitation include increased speed of recovery, positive psychological effects for the pet and owner, improved movement, increased strength, and endurance and improved biomechanics. For the veterinary cancer patient much of the rehabilitation will be for pain relief, wound healing, and postsurgical situations. With working or performance dogs the owner's goal may be to return to full performance, which may or may not be realistic depending on the pet's individual condition.

## *Assessment of Limb Function*

Limb function is evaluated using both objective and subjective joint assessments. The quality of joint motion is subjective and involves the assessment of joint biomechanics, crepitus, and pain during motion. The quantity of joint flexion and extension motion is measured using a goniometer. To measure a comfortable range of motion the joint is flexed until the first signs of discomfort and then extended. The mean of three independent measurements is used. Assessment of muscle is important in rehabilitation. Muscle mass, strength, and injury may be assessed to help evaluate progress. Limb measurements indicate limb use and muscle strength. Measurement of limb function is a valuable tool in assessing many cancer patients. Keeping assessments of limb function and muscle strength postsurgery and throughout disease progression can aid owners in making quality-of-life decisions.

Rehabilitation modalities can include therapeutic exercises and stretching, aquatic therapy, therapeutic massage and joint manipulation, the application of heat and cold, therapeutic ultrasound, electrical stimulation, low-level lasers, magnetic fields, and extracorporeal shockwaves. Treatment considerations and choice of exercise vary with the patient's stage of disease and endurance level. Veterinary oncology nurses can learn more about the uses of each modality from a variety of sources. However, they may want to spend some time with a trained veterinary physical therapist, CCRP (Certified Canine Rehabilitation Practitioner) or complete training themselves.

## Therapeutic Exercises (or Active Physical Therapy)

### Leash Walking

Leash walking is the simplest, most convenient, and most important exercise for any pet. This exercise is easy to adapt to any pet and can be easily modified as the pet improves. It also has muscular and heart-health benefits for everyone involved with minimal cost. Leash walking exercises can be performed at a variety of outdoor areas, such as sidewalks, local parks, or recreation areas. Leash walking exercises can begin shortly after surgery if there are no contraindications. Start with a slow walk at a pace comfortable for the pet. If the pace is too fast, the pet may lift the painful leg to avoid bearing weight on it. Encourage the pet to use the affected leg by praising him or her for putting the leg on the ground. In the beginning, the walks should last only 2–5 minutes two to three times daily. The exercises can be more challenging by increasing the length of time of the exercise session and increasing the speed of the walk. As the pet improves, use steeper and longer hills. Other options for increasing the benefits of the walks include walking with the dog through snow, sand, or tall grass.

### Incline/Decline Exercise

Incline and decline exercises strengthen the muscles in a pet's legs. They are easy to do and cause minimal impact on the pet's joints. An incline exercise involves walking up a hill or slope. A decline exercise involves walking down a hill or slope. When a pet walks on an incline, the back legs are exercised by moving the body forward. When the pet walks on a decline, the back legs stretch more and more weight can be put on the front legs. This reduces pain in the back legs. Start slowly with gentle inclines and declines. As the pet improves, use steeper and longer inclines and declines. You can also make the exercises more challenging by increasing the length of time you do the exercise and increasing the speed of the walk.

### Cavaletti

Cavaletti rails are horizontal poles spaced out on the ground. Cavaletti rails can also be placed horizontally at a low height. Exercises using Cavaletti rails require a pet to pick of the gastrointestinal tract; pain in some cases; aggressive glutamine uptake by tumor cells resulting in whole-body depletion of glutamine, which requires more muscle protein breakdown; obligate but inefficient glucose utilization by tumor cells; and other metabolic changes that alter nutrient processing. These are believed to be primarily mediated by cytokines, which reduce appetite, increase the metabolic rate, increase amino acid release from muscles, and mobilize fat and protein stores. Cancer cachexia results in obvious weight loss, which leads to weakness and a reduced capacity for activity that causes an obvious impact on quality of life, as well as shortened survival time (Figure 12.1). In one study, cats with cancer that were below the median for body condition scoring had a median survival time of 3.3 months compared to 16.7 months for cats above the median. Less obvious manifestations include anemia, delayed wound healing, and reduced immune function. When cancer is cured, patients regain their weight and strength and all metabolic consequences resolve.

In pets, metabolic alterations associated with cancer cachexia have been very well documented, and while some pets with cancer develop clinically evident cancer cachexia, clinically significant cancer cachexia in pets is relatively uncommon. In fact, more veterinary cancer patients struggle with obesity than with weight loss (Figure 12.2). In one study of dogs with cancer, only 4% were felt to have cachexia (as defined by a subjective scoring system); while nearly 30% were classified as overweight or obese.

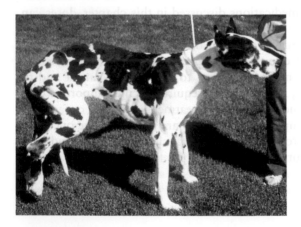

**Figure 12.1.** Severe pain from an untreated osteosarcoma of the right hindleg has led to severe cancer cachexia in this Great Dane. Pain relief (see Chapter 11) and nutritional support are vital to improve this patient's quality of life. (Courtesy of Dr. Gregory K. Ogilvie)

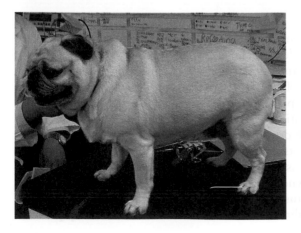

**Figure 12.2.** Obesity is more common than cachexia, particularly in canine cancer patients, and this should be taken into account when formulating a nursing plan. A few extra treats contribute to quality of life and the strength of the human-animal bond, and a little extra weight "in case they get sick" is not to be discouraged. However severe weight gain can affect the pet's quality of life.

However, when cancer cachexia does occur it undoubtedly has a substantial impact on the physical well-being and quality of life of the patient, as well as being of great concern to pet owners. This is particularly true of cats where even a small weight loss can translate into a large percentage of their body weight and be debilitating.

Nutritional support for cancer patients begins with assessment, and the nurse plays an important role in history-taking and evaluation of body condition. It is important to ask the client about the pet's appetite, regular diet, preferred foods, recent changes, any medications and supplements, and whether he or she has lost weight; it should not be assumed that an animal has not lost weight without knowing their starting point. Body weight should be recorded at every visit. Remember that changes in muscle mass are not always reflected in the body weight, especially if there is a heavy tumor burden, ascites, or edema. Therefore, physical examination for body fat stores and evidence of muscle wasting, as well as visual evaluation of body condition, are also important, although these are somewhat subjective. Use of a consistent body condition scoring system is helpful. The client's impression of the patient's body condition is also very helpful, and many clients, although not formally trained, are keen observers and can be a very reliable source of information about their pet's condition.

When nutritional support is needed, the first question is whether dietary intervention is sufficient or whether a feeding tube, or even parenteral nutrition, is needed.

Optimal dietary guidelines for patients with cancer who have a functioning gastrointestinal tract have been investigated in both humans and pets with cancer. Most importantly, the diet for all cancer patients should be highly palatable—this is critically important for quality of life as well as for nutritional support. In general, the carbohydrate content should be kept low, and in particular simple sugars should be avoided as these are not well metabolized by the host, and preferentially metabolized by tumor cells. The protein/fat balance is somewhat controversial and depends on individual factors. For most cancers that have been studied, a diet that emphasizes fat as well as protein has been found to be preferable. However, dogs with mammary cancer have been shown to have better outcomes when fed a low-fat, high-protein ration. The diet should also be complete and balanced in micronutrients (vitamins and minerals), easily digestible, and energy dense. The use of a commercially prepared food from a responsible company avoids major nutrient imbalances. The role of glutamine supplementation is well established in dogs as well as in humans with cancer. Arginine supplementation may also be useful but has not yet been studied as thoroughly. Omega-3 fatty acids have also been found to be beneficial in general for cancer patients, and supplementation (such as with fish oil capsules) is recommended for dogs not receiving a food that is already rich in these. Many committed pet owners enjoy preparing food for their pets, and this can be done safely and appropriately by following specific recipes that are available (see Figure 12.3). In addition, for pets undergoing chemotherapy, the diet should be reasonably consistent and stable, and any meat and eggs should be cooked to reduce the risk of bacterial infection.

## Gastrointestinal Supportive Medications

The first step in encouraging patients to eat as well as possible is to ensure that the gastrointestinal tract is in the best possible condition and that nausea and hyperacidity are minimized. Several types of supportive medications can assist in this.

**Ogilvie's Homemade Canine Cancer Food: A balanced homemade formula for dogs with cancer**

The following recipe will make three days worth of food for a 12-15 kilogram dog.

| Ingredients | Amount |
| --- | --- |
| Lean ground beef, fat drained | 454 grams (1 pound) |
| Rice, cooked | 227 grams (1 1/3 cups) |
| Liver, beef | 138 grams (1/3 pound) |
| Vegetable oil | 63 grams (4 ½ Tbs) |
| Fish oil | 9 grams (9x1000-mg fish oil capsules)* |
| Calcium carbonate | 3.3 grams** |
| Dicalcium phosphate*** | 2.9 grams (3/4 tsp) |
| Salt substitute (potassium chloride) | 1.9 grams (1/3 tsp) |
| Commercial Vitamin / Mineral Tablets for Dogs | |

\* Note: Owners are encouraged to feed the highest fish (or preferably docosahexaenoic acid (DHA)) oil dose tolerated by the dog.

\*\* Calcium carbonate is available as oyster shell calcium tablets or Tums® tablets (0.5 g in regular Tums, 0.75 g in Tums Extra and 1.0 g in Tums Ultra).

\*\*\* Bone meal can be used in place of dicalcium phosphate.

Directions:

Cook the rice with salt substitute added to the water. Cook the ground beef and drain the fat. Cook the liver and dice or finely chop into small pieces. Pulverize the calcium carbonate and vitamin/mineral tablets. Mix the vegetable oil, fish oil (break open capsules) and supplements with the rice and then add the cooked ground beef and liver. Mix well, cover and refrigerate. Feed approximately one-third of this mixture each day to a 25-30 pound dog. Palatability will be increased if the daily portion is heated to approximately body temperature. *Caution*: when using microwave, avoid "hot spots," which can burn the mouth.

Nutrient Profile (% dry matter basis):

| | |
| --- | --- |
| Protein | 35.3 |
| Fat | 41.6 |
| Carbohydrate | 17.8 |
| Calcium | 0.65 |
| Phosphorus | 0.54 |
| Sodium | 0.36 |
| Potassium | 0.68 |
| Magnesium | 0.05 |
| Energy | 1,989 kcal/kg as fed |

**Figure 12.3.** This diet has been developed for canine cancer patients by Dr. Gregory Ogilvie, and is a good diet for owners and their pets that enjoy home cooking. (Courtesy of Dr. Gregory Ogilvie)

## Antiemetics

For pets undergoing chemotherapy, loss of appetite may be the first sign of nausea and this should be considered before prescribing appetite stimulants. Proactive antiemetic use may solve the problem of inappetence and contribute to improved quality of life. Metoclopramide is an inexpensive, basic prophylactic antiemetic that owners can use at home from the start of chemotherapy or have on hand in case symptoms arise; it is effective for most patients. For patients who still experience nausea and vomiting, more effective antiemetics now available include maropitant, ondansetron, and dolasetron; butorphanol also has antiemetic properties and is useful in certain settings. In addition to the obvious quality-of-life benefit, effective antiemetic use also benefits the patient from a cancer management standpoint, by allowing chemotherapy to be maintained at the highest possible dose intensity.

## Gastroprotectants

Some patients are at risk for gastric ulceration either from their cancer (dogs and cats with advanced mast cell tumors may have increased levels of histamine causing gastric acid production and ulceration) or as a side effect of treatment (NSAIDs), or even from another disease process. Such patients may benefit from gastric protectants. Drugs that block histamine ($H_2$) receptors act to decrease gastric acid production, and hence reduce the risk of gastric ulceration. The most commonly used are ranitidine and famotidine. Another option to reduce gastric acid production is omeprazole; a proton pump inhibitor, which "shuts down" parietal cell production of acid very effectively. For animals that already have gastric ulceration, sucralfate can be used to bind with the ulcerated tissue and protect it from further damage while healing occurs. Sucralfate may be more effective when delivered as a slurry (rather than the tablets, which are quite large for smaller patients).

## Appetite Stimulants

The use of appetite stimulants may be appropriate for short-term support of pets experiencing a loss of appetite caused by the disease or treatment and that is expected to be self-limiting. However, their use should be carefully considered for the individual patient; often a feeding tube (below) would be a more appropriate choice. Appetite stimulants that are useful in veterinary oncology include megestrol acetate, cyproheptadine, diazepam, and mirtazapine. Cyproheptadine may be dosed every 12 hours or less frequently if inappetence is mild; if given at night it may cause erratic behavior in some patients, including vocalization and restlessness, so we suggest giving it once daily in the morning. Megestrol acetate is an effective appetite stimulant in cats, and long-term side effects are not usually a serious concern in cancer patients using it for short-term support. In humans, megestrol acetate not only improves appetite but also enhances enjoyment of food. The use of anabolic hormones is not usually rewarding, but it may be helpful in selected individual patients.

## Additional Nutritional Support

### Assisted Feeding

Hand-feeding or spoon-feeding a highly palatable, aromatic, and warmed diet may be appealing to some pets and overcome mild inappetence. (Figures 12.4–12.6) Force-feeding, on the other hand, rapidly becomes extremely stressful for both pet and owner and should be discouraged because it reduces quality of life and risks damaging the human-animal bond. For pets that are protein-calorie malnourished, increasing the frequency of feeding can help increase the overall daily intake. Finally, although reduced exercise tolerance is common in patients with cancer cachexia and these patients should not be overtaxed, some exercise is encouraged when possible to help maintain muscle mass and stimulate appetite.

### Feeding Tubes

For patients that have a functioning gut but cannot or will not maintain adequate voluntary intake, a feeding tube must be considered. Examples are pets with oral tumors or those

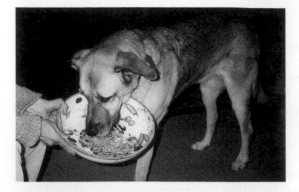

**Figure 12.4.** This dog lost considerable weight due to pain from an osteosarcoma and was inappetent on chemotherapy after amputation. Encouragement in the form of aromatic palatable foods and assisted feeding can overcome this kind of mild inappetance without the need for drugs.

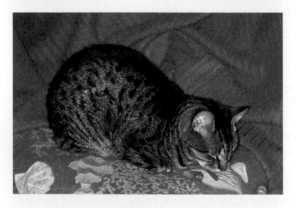

**Figure 12.5.** A febrile and inappetent cat.

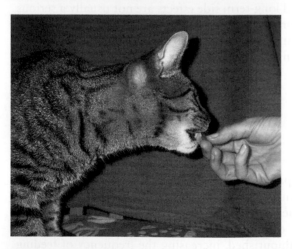

**Figure 12.6.** Hand-feeding with a highly palatable diet (smoked salmon in this instance) can overcome the mild inappetence seen in Figure 12.5.

undergoing surgery or radiotherapy of the face, or pets that have anorexia that does not respond to appetite stimulation, but no nausea or vomiting. Although the decision to place a feeding tube is quite daunting for many pet owners, once it is done many pet owners are greatly relieved to know that their pet is assured of receiving adequate nutrition without a struggle and find that their pets are feeling better. An added advantage of a feeding tube is that it eases administration of oral medications. Several different types of feeding tubes are used, and the relative advantages and disadvantages are summarized below.

Nasoesophageal tubes are placed through the nares and into the distal esophagus (rather than into the stomach, to avoid gastric reflux). This is the only type of feeding tube that can be placed without anesthesia and without creating a stoma, so it a good choice in critically ill patients that would present a high anesthetic risk or who are expected to require nutritional support for a relatively short time. This is also the least expensive feeding tube. The major disadvantage is that because of the small size of the tube, only a liquid diet can be used. Risks include vomiting, esophagitis, and aspiration pneumonia. Also, some patients are annoyed by the tube in their nose and around their eyes, and these tubes are not a good choice for patients with severe facial or head sensitivity, such as after extensive surgery.

Esophagostomy tubes are placed under anesthesia through a stoma created into the esophagus in the neck. This is a relatively inexpensive type of feeding tube. It has the advantage of being less annoying, particularly to cats, and the slightly larger tube can accommodate feeding gruel as well as liquid. It is a less complex placement procedure and less costly to place than a gastrostomy tube. Again, vomiting, esophagitis, and aspiration pneumonia are risks with these tubes.

Gastrostomy tubes are placed under anesthesia with or without endoscopy depending on the tube, creating a stoma through the abdominal wall. This larger tube can accommodate gruel as well as liquid, and can remain in place and functional for very long periods of time. Feeding needs to be carefully managed in some patients to avoid triggering vomiting.

Jejunostomy tubes are the only choice for enteral nutrition in patients who have small intestinal function, but also have frequent vomiting, no gag reflex, or no gastric function; these tubes can even be used in some comatose patients. However, they are considerably more complex to place and use than the other types of tubes, and they require small frequent feedings or continuous slow feeding of liquid food only. The tubes can clog, and diets need to be very carefully managed to avoid causing vomiting or diarrhea, hyperglycemia or hypoglycemia, or electrolyte imbalances.

## Parenteral Feeding

Enteral feeding is chosen over parenteral feeding whenever possible. Parenteral nutrition is much more complex and costly, and it carries a much higher risk of complications. Further, the cells lining the gastrointestinal tract are starved by long-term lack of direct food intake, resulting in atrophy, loss of enzyme activity, loss of local immune function, and loss of normal microflora, all of which further debilitate the gastrointestinal tract and complicate the return to normal feeding. Nonetheless, there are situations where the gastrointestinal tract is totally nonfunctional for a period of time or must be totally rested (e.g., pancreatitis, ileus, ongoing vomiting/diarrhea). Luckily, such cases are rare, but when they are identified, parenteral nutrition is required.

Total parental nutrition (TPN) is used to meet all of a patient's nutritional needs. TPN is a highly specialized process and should be used only where 24-hour nursing care is available. TPN must be given through a dedicated central venous catheter, and aseptic procedure must be extremely strict, in both preparation of solutions and administration, to minimize the infection risk. TPN feeding solutions include dextrose, amino acids, lipids, vitamins and minerals, and electrolytes; the precise formulation is individualized according to the patient's specific requirements. Fluid therapy may be needed in addition. Feeding must be initiated and concluded gradually and done with close monitoring for hyperlipidemia, hyperglycemia, azotemia, and electrolyte imbalances.

A slightly less aggressive option that can be used for shorter time periods is partial parenteral nutrition (PPN). PPN uses amino acid solutions with electrolytes to minimize protein malnutrition. PPN can be given through a peripheral catheter, but close monitoring is still required, and the infection risk is still higher than with intravenous fluids, so asepsis must be strict.

## Strategies for Gastrointestinal Supportive Care in Critically Ill Cancer Patients

The principles of supportive care for unwell patients starting chemotherapy are illustrated well by the strategies used for dogs with substage b (unwell) lymphoma (Figure 12.7). In one study, of 40 dogs with lymphoma eating normally before diagnosis, nearly 90% achieved complete remission; of 52 inappetent dogs, fewer than 60% achieved complete remission. Of dogs that can achieve a complete remission, those that are inappetent at entry have shorter overall disease control; inappetent dogs had median remission times of 5 months compared with 12 months for dogs that were eating well. Supportive care can improve both the remission rate and survival as well as quality of life for the patient.

Dogs with lymphoma in substage b (particularly anorexia and other gastrointestinal signs) should be given intravenous fluid therapy (maintenance × 1.5), broad-spectrum antibiotics (cefazolin or enrofloxacin (see Appendix 4)), and gastrointestinal prophylaxis (metoclopramide, omeprazole, and bland food diet). This supportive care should be continued for at least 4 days after chemotherapy is started and preferably for a week. Dogs can be treated at home with oral medication as soon as they are self-supporting, and antibiotics and prophylactic metoclopramide are continued *for the first 3 weeks of the*

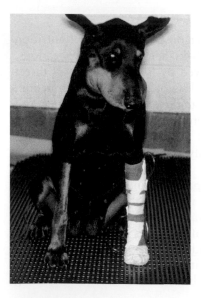

**Figure 12.7.** This very ill dog with lymphoma will benefit from fluid therapy support and antinausea medications. Although chemotherapy remains the treatment most likely to extend her survival, supportive care means she is more likely to respond.

*protocol.* Appetite stimulants can also be used in this setting if there is no vomiting. Some patients appear to recover well in the first week and then deteriorate again in the second or third week after starting chemotherapy for lymphoma. Continuing supportive care with antibiotics and metoclopramide during this time helps ensure that the patient does as well as possible and that its owners don't become discouraged. It is also important to keep the chemotherapy at the highest intensity possible while supporting the patient; however, judicious use of chemotherapy breaks to allow recovery is also important.

Similar to dogs, cats in substage b have a worse prognosis than those that are well before starting chemotherapy for lymphoma. Due to their small size, supportive care is even more important in cats than in dogs. Cats may lose a large percentage of their body weight in even as short a period as a week, and loss of more than 5% of their weight should be considered unacceptable. Antiemetics and appetite stimulants may be appropriate in addition to good general nursing care in order to improve nutritional status if chemotherapy is used; a feeding tube should be considered for patients refractory to these interventions.

## Supportive Care for Gastrointestinal Side Effects of Chemotherapy

For animals that are not sick when beginning treatment, gastrointestinal side effects of chemotherapy are less likely but still a possibility. Vomiting is not usually a significant problem for most dogs and cats receiving chemotherapy; however, antiemetics given prophylactically for 4 to 5 days each time doxorubicin (and for some animals, vincristine) is given will reduce the risk of nausea. As with pain, it is easier to prevent nausea than to treat it, so prophylactic antiemetic use is appropriate. Vincristine may result in intestinal ileus in cats and less commonly in dogs. Prokinetic drugs such as metoclopramide may act to prevent or reverse this toxicity. The use of prophylactic metoclopramide is recommended by some practitioners to reduce the risk of inappetence due to vincristine and also doxorubicin (perhaps by central action to reduce nausea). In the prophylactic setting, treatment is started at the time of chemotherapy and continued for 4 to 5 days. In addition, from the day of treatment with doxorubicin (if that drug is used), administration of Tribrissen (trimethoprim-sulphadiazine) for 14 days markedly reduces the likelihood of gastrointestinal toxicity (vomiting or diarrhea), hospitalization, and reduced quality of life. The effect may be due to reduced bacterial translocation in damaged intestinal epithelial layers.

For any pet receiving chemotherapy, the diet should be stable, but this is especially important for pets prone to diarrhea or experiencing diarrhea as a side effect. When a pet has cancer, owners often feel giving as many treats as possible will help improve their quality of life. Although such an approach should not be discouraged in principle, consideration should be given to the possibility for the patient to develop other problems such as diarrhea, pancreatitis, or significant obesity. Prophylactic absorbents such as kaolin and pectin are often helpful for dogs experiencing diarrhea on chemotherapy. In addition, a bland diet should be offered, and if diarrhea persists, and causes such as parasitism in these often immunosuppressed patients have been eliminated, sulfasalazine or metronidazole may reduce the severity. Patients experiencing severe diarrhea can become dehydrated and may require fluid support. If diarrhea is hemorrhagic broad-spectrum antibiotics should be given because of the risk of bacterial translocation in potentially immunosuppressed patients.

# Further Reading

Baez JL, et al. 2007. A prospective investigation of the prevalence and prognostic significance of weight loss and changes in body condition in feline cancer patients. *J Feline Med Surg* 9:411–417.

Benchaoui HA, et al. 2007. Efficacy of maropitant for preventing vomiting associated with motion sickness in dogs. *Vet Rec* 161:444–447.

Chretin JD, et al. 2007. Prophylactic trimethoprim-sulfadiazine during chemotherapy in dogs with lymphoma and osteosarcoma: a double-blind, placebo-controlled study. *J Vet Intern Med* 21(1):141–148.

Hickman MA, et al. 2008. Safety, pharmacokinetics and use of the novel NK-1 receptor antagonist maropitant (CereniaTM) for the prevention of emesis and motion sickness in cats. *J Vet Pharmacol Therap* 31(3):220–229.

Michel KE, et al. 2004. Evaluation of body condition and weight loss in dogs presented to a veterinary oncology service. *J Vet Intern Med* 18:692–695.

Morrison-Collister KE, et al. 2004. A combination chemotherapy protocol with MOPP and CCNU consolidation (Tufts VELCAP-SC) for the treatment of canine lymphoma. *Vet Compar Oncol* 1:180–190.

Ogilvie GK. 2000. Dolasetron: a new option for nausea and vomiting. *J Am Anim Hosp Assoc* 36:481–483.

Sedlacek HS, et al. 2008. Comparative efficacy of maropitant and selected drugs in preventing emesis induced by centrally or peripherally acting emetogens in dogs. *J Vet Pharmacol Ther* 31:533–537.

# Hematologic Support

13

*Note:* For the antibiotics discussed in this chapter, doses can be found in Appendix 4.

As discussed previously, the bone marrow is one of the most sensitive organs to chemotherapy, so hematologic side effects are common. In addition, many cancers have a direct or indirect (paraneoplastic) effect on bone marrow function. Thus, hematologic supportive care is often needed for our patients.

## CBC Changes Associated with Cancer Treatment

The cancer treatment most likely to cause hematologic changes in pets is chemotherapy. All anticancer chemotherapy drugs have the potential to produce adverse side effects. However, the side effects that can occur in pets are usually not as severe or as long lasting as those that occur in humans due to the lower doses used. Most clients are pleasantly surprised at how well their pets feel during chemotherapy. Despite the lower doses and lower risks of toxicity, some toxicity may occur, primarily following the first time a patient receives a chemotherapy drug and before the dose has been "individualized" for that patient. Of these toxicities, neutropenia is the one that is most likely to be life-threatening, due to the increased risk of sepsis.

*Myelosuppression* is a general term applied to the toxic effects of chemotherapy on the bone marrow. The most chemosensitive cells in the bone marrow are the proliferating progenitors and precursors, which are starting to commit to a particular lineage but are still immature. The more differentiated cells form a nonproliferating pool of maturing cells that will be unaffected by chemotherapy and will provide mature cells for a period of days. Like the maturing cells, hematopoietic stem cells are largely nonproliferating and so are relatively resistant to chemotherapy toxicity. However, they are stimulated to divide by the loss of proliferating precursor cells, and they rapidly replace the lost cells so that cytopenias following chemotherapy rarely last more than several days. This also has implications for the interval between administrations of myelosuppressive drugs. If these

**Table 13.1.** Myelosuppressive effects of chemotherapeutic agents used in veterinary medicine

| Highly Myelosuppressive | Moderately Myelosuppressive | Mildly Myelosuppressive |
|---|---|---|
| Doxorubicin | Melphalan | L-asparaginase[a] |
| Vinblastine | Chlorambucil | Vincristine[a] |
| Cyclophosphamide | 5-Fluorouracil | Bleomycin |
| Lomustine (CCNU) | Methotrexate | Corticosteroids |
| Actinomycin-D | Procarbazine | |
| Mitoxantrone | Cisplatin | |
| Carboplatin | | |

[a]More pronounced myelosuppression can occur if these two drugs are administered concurrently.

drugs are given when the stem cell pool is dividing (i.e., soon after the previous administration), severe prolonged myelosuppression due to stem cell destruction may occur. For this reason, the usual interval between myelosuppressive drug administrations is 2 to 3 weeks. Some drugs (such as lomustine and carboplatin) may have delayed or prolonged nadirs, and dosing intervals are longer for these drugs. The relative likelihood of causing myelosuppression varies between drugs (Table 13.1) and between species.

Although myelosuppression does disrupt erythropoiesis, anemia as a direct chemotherapy side effect is rarely of clinical significance in veterinary oncology, because of the relatively long lifespan of red blood cells (120 days in dogs, 70 days in cats). When it does occur it is usually only in long-term chemotherapy patients, and it tends to be a low-grade anemia with a gradual onset. Acute anemia in a chemotherapy patient should prompt consideration of blood loss or hemolysis.

Thrombocytopenia occasionally may occur as a direct chemotherapy side effect, although usually it is not dose-limiting. Although it can follow treatment with any myelosuppressive drug, it is most likely to be significant after treatment with carboplatin or lomustine. Chemotherapy-related thrombocytopenia rarely causes clinical signs; however, at counts of less than 50,000/μl the risk of bleeding increases and the technician/nurse should be alert to petechiation, ecchymoses, or mucosal bleeding. Myelosuppressive chemotherapy should generally not be administered if the platelet count is less than 100,000/μl.

Sepsis due to chemotherapy or cancer-related neutropenia is one of the more common emergencies in veterinary cancer medicine, but it is usually preventable through judicious monitoring and appropriate supportive care. In addition, caregivers should be educated about the early clinical signs of neutropenia and thrombocytopenia induced by cancer treatment so that they can assist in early detection and seek immediate treatment. The risk of developing neutropenic sepsis is probably less than 5% in veterinary patients, but because dogs may hide their symptoms until late in the disease, the condition of sepsis may be quite advanced when first recognized and requires prompt, emergency intervention. Timely treatment can make the difference between life and death for these patients.

The most important risk factor for sepsis is the *absolute neutrophil count* and it is important to attend to this rather than the total white cell count or the relative (%) neutrophil count, both of which can be highly misleading.

Knowing the myelosuppressive potential for chemotherapy drugs being administered, and having an estimate of the time that the neutrophil (not just total white cell count) nadir (lowest count) will occur, allows the cancer treatment team to plan monitoring blood counts and to administer prophylactic antibiotics, if that approach is chosen. Chemotherapy agents vary as to how myelosuppressive they are and therefore how likely they are to cause neutropenia and hence increase the risk of sepsis (Table 13.1).

The timing of the neutrophil nadir also varies from drug to drug. The neutrophil nadir occurs 7 to 10 days after administration for most chemotherapeutics, and for consistency a CBC is collected 7 days after administration. This is done to assess both the immediate risk of sepsis, and whether the future dosage of that drug needs to be changed. The aim is to have a segmented neutrophil count at the nadir of between 1000/µl and 3000/µl. The nadir is usually of short duration at the doses used in veterinary medicine, recovering to normal within 48–72 hours. Some drugs may cause a "delayed" neutrophil nadir; for example, carboplatin may cause a nadir 2 or even 3 weeks after administration in cats and in some dogs, and recovery to normal may be further delayed, particularly in cats. It is important to know the expected nadir time and severity for each drug administered, in each species, and to be familiar with factors that could cause alterations in chemotherapy drug metabolism that could increase the risk of myelosuppression (e.g., reduced renal clearance may exacerbate the myelosuppressive effects of carboplatin).

Prophylactic antibiotic therapy is often recommended for patients receiving myelosuppressive chemotherapy as a method of reducing the risk of sepsis. The costs of prophylactic treatment may be weighed against the decreased risk of morbidity due to sepsis, as well as decreased risk of hospitalization and costs associated with it. Some oncologists recommend use of trimethoprim sulfa (unless contraindicated) as a prophylactic measure in any dog receiving a myelosuppressive chemotherapy agent for the first time (until the nadir neutrophil count is known) because this drug is relatively inexpensive, orally administered, and has little negative effect on gastrointestinal flora. This approach has been shown to reduce morbidity and hospitalization in dogs treated with doxorubicin chemotherapy for osteosarcoma or lymphoma.

Careful reading of the hematology report, both at baseline pretreatment evaluation and during treatment, can provide key information that will allow the cancer treatment team to modify treatment for optimal management of each patient and direct further diagnostics when needed. Although many anticancer chemotherapeutics have myelosuppressive potential, at the doses used in veterinary medicine most neutropenia caused by cancer treatment can be managed, resulting in minimal impact on the patient's quality of life. It is important to be aware of the variation in myelosuppressive potential and timing of the individual drugs being used. Detailed education of caregivers in combination with careful monitoring and prompt appropriate therapy when indicated will result in good outcomes for the great majority of neutropenic chemotherapy patients.

## Practical Tip

If you need a complete blood count before giving a myelosuppressive agent (to make sure the neutrophil count is above 3000/µl) and it needs to be sent to an outside laboratory, consider collecting it the day before and then arranging the chemotherapy appointment for a time when you know that the results will be back.

## Managing Neutropenic Patients

### How to Manage Mild (Grade 1) or Moderate (Grade 2) Neutropenia

For most chemotherapy patients the neutrophil count at the expected nadir is between normal and 1500/µl (grade 1) or between 1500/µl and 1000/µl (grade 2). At this level the risk of complicating illness is low, but because the time of the true nadir is not known for an individual patient, prophylactic antibiotics should be considered. Good choices of broad-spectrum orally administered antibiotics include trimethoprim-sulpha combinations for most dogs, or enrofloxacin. Enrofloxacin is also a good choice in cats but orbifloxacin appears to cause less nausea. Prior to the next dose of myelosuppressive chemotherapy, rechecking the CBC should be considered and the next drug should not be administered unless the neutrophil count is above 3000/µl.

For animals experiencing mild or moderate neutropenia, the dosage of the chemotherapy drug causing that effect does **not** need to be changed the next time the drug is administered unless recovery is delayed requiring the next treatment to be postponed.

### How to Manage Marked (Grade 3) Neutropenia

For some animals the myelosuppressive effects of chemotherapy may be more pronounced; in these pets the neutrophil count may be between 1000/µl and 500/µl (grade 3) following chemotherapy. At this level the risk of complicating illness is much higher, although most animals still will not experience sepsis as long as they are receiving prophylactic antibiotics. Antibiotics should be continued, or started in pets that are not receiving them. A full examination of the patient should be performed, but the pet should **not** be hospitalized unless parenteral care is needed because this may increase the risk for sepsis. Owners should be instructed to check the temperature (preferably rectal) at least twice a day and contact the veterinary clinic if it is above normal on two occasions 30 minutes apart. Additionally, any signs of illness (lethargy, anorexia, vomiting, diarrhea) should be reported promptly, and the patient treated as an emergency. Prior to the next dose of myelosuppressive chemotherapy, another CBC should be collected and the next drug should not be administered unless the neutrophil count is above 3000/µl.

For animals experiencing moderate neutropenia, the dosage of the chemotherapy drug causing that effect should be reduced by 25% for all subsequent doses of **that drug**, and a CBC should be collected at the expected nadir after administering the reduced dose of that drug.

### How to Manage Severe (Grade 4) Neutropenia

Rarely the myelosuppressive effects of chemotherapy may be marked; in these pets the neutrophil count is below 500/µl following chemotherapy. At this level the risk of complicating illness is very high, and some animals will become septic even if they are receiving prophylactic antibiotics; these are very delicate patients. A full examination of the patient should be performed, but, again, the pet should not be hospitalized unless there is a fever or other signs of illness, and parenteral supportive care is needed. Owners should be instructed to check the temperature (preferably rectal) at least twice a day, and contact the veterinary clinic if it is above normal on 2 occasions 30 minutes apart. Additionally, any signs of illness (lethargy, anorexia, vomiting, diarrhea) should be reported promptly and the patient treated as an emergency. Prior to the next dose of any myelosuppressive chemotherapy another CBC should be collected and the next drug should not be administered unless the neutrophil count is above 3000/µl.

For animals experiencing severe (grade 4) neutropenia, the dosage of the chemotherapy drug causing that effect should be reduced by 25% for all subsequent doses of **that drug**; a CBC should be collected at the expected nadir after administering the drug at a dose reduction.

## Triage for Potentially Septic Patients

Knowing that a patient has received a myelosuppressive chemotherapy drug, and when the expected nadir of that drug will be, will help the oncology nurse in triaging the patient for further intervention. If, for example, a dog that has received doxorubicin the previous day has bloody stools, this is unlikely to be due to sepsis (too early for myelosuppression to be seen), and more likely to be due to gastrointestinal damage from the doxorubicin (most common 2 to 4 days after treatment). If the same signs were present in a dog that had received doxorubicin 7 days previously, that patient is expected to be neutropenic, and is at great risk of sepsis. However, no patient can be diagnosed remotely, and the triage procedure should be the same in both scenarios.

Assessment of the patient's hemodynamic status is mandatory; the hemodynamic derangements of septic shock are characterized by arterial hypotension, peripheral vasodilatation, hypovolemia from capillary leakage, and the development of myocardial depression. Septic shock represents failure of the circulatory system to maintain adequate delivery of oxygen and other nutrients to tissues, causing cellular and then organ dysfunction. Prompt intervention to restore circulation will be life saving in these patients. You should ensure adequate hemodynamic and respiratory support; identify and ascertain the extent of any organ dysfunction (blood work and urinalysis); and, based on that, develop an overall treatment plan (see more in Chapters 17 and 18).

One logical step to minimize the risk for sepsis for pets with severe neutropenia is to minimize the administration of immunosuppressive drugs, especially corticosteroids, except when needed for treatment of the cancer. Risk for catheter-induced sepsis in hospitalized patients can be minimized by placing a new catheter in a new site every 2 to 3 days. Strict aseptic procedures should be used, especially with animals that are myelosuppressed. The duration of hospitalization should be limited whenever possible to limit exposure to antibiotic-resistant bacteria.

If sepsis is suspected, prompt antibiotic therapy (within 8 hours of presentation) is warranted based on the most likely type(s) of infection (most sepsis in chemotherapy patients is gram-negative enterobacteria); studies in animals with septic shock indicate that mortality can directly relate to time delay in antibiotics.

Canine recombinant granulocyte colony stimulating factor (G-CSF) may increase cell numbers and enhance neutrophil function. Human recombinant G-CSF is commercially available; however, long-term use may induce antibody formation to the protein, which can cause a paradoxical neutropenia. Whether these drugs improve outcome in patients that already have neutropenia and therefore already have maximal stimulation of their endogenous G-CSF is controversial. Most neutropenic patients recover rapidly without G-CSF administration, and the rapid recovery observed after exogenous administration may be due to endogenous CSFs rather than the treatment. In human patients, trials in febrile neutropenic patients have provided conflicting results. Although neutrophil recovery times are faster with CSF and antibiotic therapy, duration of hospitalization may not be reduced except in patients receiving less myelosuppressive chemotherapy treatments.

It is our opinion that G-CSF has a role in prevention of severe myelosuppression after an inadvertent overdose of a myelosuppressive chemotherapy agent. In that situation, treatment should be started within 48 hours (but not before 24 hours) of the overdose. The use of human recombinant CSFs in febrile neutropenic patients following standard-dose chemotherapy may benefit some animals considered to be at high risk, but routine use adds unnecessary expense and prolonged administration should be avoided.

## Further Reading

Chretin JD, et al. 2007. Prophylactic trimethoprim-sulfadiazine during chemotherapy in dogs with lymphoma and osteosarcoma: a double-blind, placebo-controlled study. *J Vet Intern Med* 21(1):141–148.

Ravaud A, et al. 1998. Granulocyte-macrophage colony-stimulating factor in patients with neutropenic fever is potent after low-risk but not after high-risk neutropenic chemotherapy regimens: results of a randomized phase III trial. *J Clin Oncol* 16:2930–2936.

Veterinary Co-operative Oncology Group. 2004. Common terminology criteria for adverse events (VCOG-CTCAE) following chemotherapy or biological antineoplastic therapy in dogs and cats v1.0. *Vet Comp Oncol* 2:195–213.

# Euthanasia and End-of-Life Patient Care

Although being a veterinary technician/nurse can often be an uplifting experience, one of the most challenging aspects is that many of your patients will not be cured of their cancer, and for many of these patients euthanasia will eventually be performed. Often this will occur after you have been working with the patient and client for a long time. Some owners will not accept euthanasia under any circumstances, and for these pets, discussions about hospice home care is very important to ensure that the pet is as comfortable as possible.

The best time to discuss euthanasia will vary from patient to patient and client to client, but certainly if the caregiver brings up the subject, it should be discussed to whatever level seems comfortable. For some clients, such a discussion can take place at the first visit, when treatment options are discussed.

Many owners ask how they will know "when is the right time" to euthanize their pet. For such owners, it is a good idea for them to make a list of the positive aspects of their pet's life at a time before treatment has started, and before the cancer is advanced. This can be life-affirming and may also act as a baseline for future assessments of the impact of the cancer and treatment on quality of life, as well as a signal that the time for euthanasia is approaching.

Most clients want to be present during the euthanasia process. The ideal place for euthanasia may be dictated by the pet's medical condition. Ideally, euthanasia may be performed at home. This poses logistic problems and may be possible only if the pet visits the veterinary clinic for an intravenous catheter to be placed, and a later visit to the home scheduled by the veterinarian and nurse. A compassionate veterinary technician/nurse can make the difference between a home euthanasia going very well and it being an unsettling experience for the owner. Gentle but firm patient restraint when needed can help the veterinarian focus on the process and ensure all technical procedures go well; this also allows the owners to focus on their pet. If home euthanasia is not an option, a secluded comfortable location should be provided. If a garden area is available, this is a good choice for some clients; if not, try to identify a room that will allow the tearful client to exit privately (and not walk through a waiting room full of healthy pets and their owners).

The client is not the only one who will be affected by euthanasia, and it is important to acknowledge that every member of the veterinary oncology team is likely to be impacted by the loss of a patient. Although it is a priority for the caregiver and family to say goodbye prior to and after euthanasia, it may be important for the veterinary team as well; take time to do this. More discussion of the emotional aspects of euthanasia can be found in Chapters 15 and 16.

Some owners will wonder whether children should be involved in the decision to perform euthanasia. Excluding children or making up stories (e.g., "Fudge ran away"; or "Chippy has gone to sleep") may only lead to confusion and misinterpretation of future events. An open and honest discussion with children is imperative. They should also be allowed the chance to say goodbye to their pet.

Some owners ask whether another pet can be present. There may be some be benefit to other pets being allowed to see and sniff the patient after death and having "closure." It is important to remind owners that other pets may not respond with what they interpret as displays of grief, and they may not appear to even notice the dead companion. In such circumstances, one has to rely on the owner's feeling that some connection has been made between the departed pet and the live pet. For surviving pets that appear to be having difficulty adjusting to the death of a pet, consultation with a veterinary behaviorist may be appropriate and helpful.

Many owners might have uncertainty about what to do with their pet's remains and it might be confusing and frightening for them to consider. The options should be presented prior to euthanasia, and where health codes permit, the options of burial, cremation with return of ashes, or general cremation (no remains returned) should be offered. If burial or cremation is considered, a choice of coffins or urns may be important to some clients. Ideally, these decisions can be made in advance of euthanasia, but for some clients, the final choice and details may not be possible until after euthanasia. Some owners like to collect a keepsake of their pet by clipping some hair or taking paw prints or photographs.

## The Euthanasia Procedure

The following steps outline the euthanasia procedure:

1.  For many clients this is the most important moment they will ever spend with you. It is very important to give them your full attention and never rush this very significant event. If necessary, other staff in the practice should be discreetly made aware what is happening so that they can help to "protect" the nurse and veterinarian involved from interruption.
2.  Remember to maintain professional conduct during this emotional time, but this should not suggest that sadness or tears from the veterinary staff are ever unprofessional.
3.  Most veterinary clinics ask their clients to sign an informed consent for euthanasia. This should be done before the clients say their final goodbyes.
4.  Identify the preferred location, which can include the owner as well as children, friends, and family animals if they wish to be involved. Allow some time for the owner to be with the pet before and after euthanasia. Make sure tissues are available.

5. Draw up the appropriate amount of euthanasia solution (a Luer Lock syringe is ideal because the solution can be "sticky" causing the syringe to dislodge) as well as two saline flushes. Place the syringes out of sight when entering the room, but keep them in an easily accessible spot for the veterinarian to reach when the time is right.

6. Preplace an intravenous catheter with a rubber-tipped plug. We prefer a catheter in the back leg (the saphenous vein is ideal in dogs) because this will allow the pet to lie in lateral recumbency or to sit upright while the caregiver can be seated near the patient's head without obstruction. The catheter plug should be secure but visible and accessible without the need to remove bandages.

7. Some veterinary health care teams like to premedicate with a tranquilizer; make sure this is discussed with the owners, because they may prefer to have their pet remain fully interactive until the last possible minute.

8. Even when an owner has had a pet euthanatized before, it is helpful to review some of what will happen; remember that owners are often distraught and may need reminding.

9. Remind owners how fast the process of euthanasia is, once the injection starts. Reemphasize that the euthanasia solution is an anesthetic that is in very concentrated form. Euthanasia solution will give the pet a short period of peaceful anesthesia after which the heart and brain functions will cease. Remind them that when human patients have an anesthetic, they often cannot count backward from 10 before they lose consciousness; this emphasizes the speed of the process.

10. Remind them, that after death, the pet's eyes may not close. In addition, there may be loss of bladder and bowel control due to muscle relaxation. A blanket placed over the lower half of the patient will prevent the owner being distracted by such an event. Also, some animals will twitch or even take breaths (these can be "agonal" or noisy); advise owners that this is a normal reaction as blood flow ceases. It does not mean the patient is conscious or in pain, or distressed in any way.

11. Before the veterinarian starts injecting, check again with the owners to see whether they are ready.

12. When the owner is ready, the syringes should be retrieved, but preferably kept from direct view (the blanket over the hind quarters is good for this too). While the catheter is flushed (tell the owners this is the flush) gently restrain the leg containing the catheter. After the euthanasia is performed, allow the owner room and solitude (if needed) to say proper goodbyes and to start the process of grieving. More information about this can be found in Chapters 15 and 16. Some owners may not want to be alone, but still be near their pet, and to tell you stories; this is also fine, and time should always be set aside by the nurse for this eventuality, particularly in a busy practice where the veterinarian may have to attend to other patients.

13. Many veterinary clinics do not have clients paying the bill at this time but prefer instead to mail them the charges at a later date. This is not always feasible in some areas of the practice such as emergency; however oncology clients are usually very well established.

If an owner decides not to be present for euthanasia, that decision should be supported as well. It is still appropriate to offer an explanation of the process, in case the owner changes his or her mind, and so that there is no mystery that could later prove disquieting. Under these circumstances (when the owner is not present), the veterinary nurse may be the person most familiar with the patient, and the nurse's compassion is even more important.

It is rewarding to many veterinarians and nurses to contact the client later after euthanasia. Cards, letters, or flowers can be sent by everyone involved and can be important not only for the client but for closure for the entire team as well. Adding a picture of the patient to a scrapbook or a bulletin board of beloved pets may also be of value in memorializing your patients. There are also several veterinary nonprofit organizations that offer memorial donation programs in which veterinarians can make donations in memory of deceased patients (sometimes they can specifically be directed toward cancer research, for example), and the clients will receive an acknowledgment letter. This is often greatly appreciated by clients.

## When Euthanasia Is Not Wanted

As mentioned above, some owners do not wish their pet to be euthanatized, and the reasons should not be questioned by the veterinary team. In such situations, the owner should be instructed as to how to provide the most comfortable hospice care possible. The goal of hospice care is to help pets that are dying have peace, comfort, and dignity. The caregivers try to control pain and other symptoms so a patient can remain as alert and comfortable as possible while surrounded by their loved ones. During this time, nutrition and pain control are very important (see Chapters 11 and 12). Remind owners that if the patient's condition or the owner's decision changes, so can the care that the veterinary oncology team provides, including euthanasia.

# Section 5

## Support for Pet Owners and Caregivers

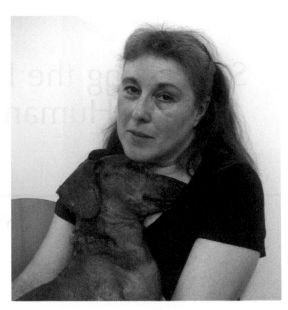

**Figure 15.1.** Owners with animals that have cancer may be confused and sad. Their bond should be recognized and supported by the veterinary cancer care team.

only care for animals but also be mindful of the emotions of the owner. As pet ownership continues to increase, many animals are considered an integral part of families. Some studies suggest that a growing number of companion animals are considered surrogate children, and that the loss of a pet could be equivalent to the grief experienced following the loss of a child. Other literature questions the tendency to relate human-animal relationships to human-human relationships and warns that this can pathologize and diminish the understanding of this relationship. Veterinary workers should be aware that the bond between animals and humans is unique and should be understood on its own terms (Figure 15.1). As workers become more experienced in the field they will come to a better understanding of the different forms human-animal relationships can take.

The role of a pet in a family can vary from guard dog to mice catcher to beloved companion or child. The pet begins to become a member of the family at the point of selection or entry into the home, and its role develops with time. Pets can provide unconditional love and a barrier against loneliness and fulfill the human need to be needed.

Assuming knowledge of a pet-owner relationship based on previous experience, or other factors such as age or social or cultural circumstances should be avoided. Just as the animal-human bond is unique, every pet-owner bond is different. It is important to recognize and acknowledge the role of the animal in the home in order to form a context for intervention and to appreciate the implications of a cancer diagnosis. A 2000 study of pet owners who had recently had a pet die showed that 82% of participants believed that the degree of attachment they had for their animal was the determining factor in the amount of grief they were experiencing (Adams et al. 2000). Taking the time to explore the pet-owner bond with clients will be valuable when working with them on an ongoing basis.

## Grief and Loss

Grief reactions are experienced in the context of all major life changes, such as divorce, changing locations, and the death of a loved one. No expression of grief is "right" or "wrong." There is considerable literature available on grief and loss theories. In 1970 Kubler-Ross famously identified five stages of grief: denial, anger, bargaining, depression, and acceptance. More recent literature redefines this somewhat by describing a number of different phases that people may go through, often returning to a phase many times. Herbert (1997) describes four phases of uncomplicated grieving: numbness, yearning, disorganization and despair, and reorganization.

Generally the grieving process starts at the point of a cancer diagnosis. Initially the grief may be related to the loss of health, guilt over not recognizing symptoms, concern over lifestyle changes, and disbelief that a previously healthy animal has become unwell. If the patient becomes terminal the owner begins to grieve for the impending loss and begins to consider difficult issues such as euthanasia and pain management, telling other family members, and preparing for the loss. After a pet's death the owner mourns the loss of companionship. At any time through the cancer journey the owner may be experiencing a myriad of emotions.

Some of the reactions that may be experienced by owners are

1. *Shock.* This can mean feeling emotionally numb and a refusal to believe what is happening. This is frequently a person's first reaction to upsetting news because it can form a protective barrier of sorts as the person attempts to process or make sense of the information. It is not unusual for an owner to require information to be repeated at some stage after their initial consultation because of inability to remember what was said at the time.
2. *Anger.* People may direct anger at themselves or others. Often caregivers and health professionals will be targets of anger as people try to find somebody to blame. People may show signs of irritation, agitation, or even aggression. Anger is not uncommon at any stage of the grieving process.
3. *Sadness.* Extreme and overwhelming sadness is not uncommon. People can become listless and withdrawn, and cry easily.
4. *Bargaining.* Many people may try to think of how they could have handled a situation differently—for example, asking, "What if I'd taken him to be assessed sooner?" Some attempt to make a deal or bargain, such as, "If I pay him more attention everything will be okay."
5. *Guilt.* Guilt can be an overwhelming and often irrational feeling. Many people feel guilty after a bereavement whether or not there was anything they could have done differently. People will question the actions and decisions they made and wonder what would have happened if they had done something differently.
6. *Yearning.* This is characterized by an intense longing for the lost pet. Some people experience physical pain such as aching arms as they long to hold their pet again.
7. *Physical reactions.* This may include changes in appetite, sleep disturbances, fatigue, nausea, tightness in the chest, headaches, and digestive problems. It is also possible for a bereaved person to suffer from auditory or visual hallucinations, and believe they have seen or heard their pet after he or she has died.

8.   *Anxiety and depression.* It is important to be aware of the difference between "normal" grief reactions and clinical mental health disorders. It is possible for a bereaved person to develop a depressive disorder or anxiety that requires medical and/or psychological intervention. An existing condition may also be exacerbated. If a person is showing signs of extreme depression or suicidality or is experiencing prolonged and severe grief reactions, referral to an appropriate health professional is suggested.

## When a Pet Is Dying

A 2007 study showed that 30% of participants experienced severe grief in the months following the death of a pet. The risk factors identified for grief were level of attachment of the owner to the pet, euthanasia, societal attitudes toward pet death, and professional support from the veterinary team.

## *How Can the Nurse Help?*

The veterinary team members "must be mindful that their approach to caring for a client whose pet has died has the potential to alleviate or aggravate grief." Health workers should take the time to consider what would be most helpful to them in a crisis. Kindness, compassion, and a respectful attitude are very important. Every client is unique, and it is important that the team tailor its response to suit the individual. The following sections discuss some basic skills that the health care team can employ.

### Compassion

By showing concern and a caring manner, staff can immediately convey a sense to clients that they are in a supportive environment. A smile, a patient manner, and a kind tone of voice will put clients at ease and increase their sense of being understood.

### Validate and Normalize

The veterinary team can show by their words and manner that a client's feelings are legitimate and understandable. Allow owners to speak about how they are feeling and show an acceptance and understanding of these feelings. Let people know that others have felt the same way in the past.

### Encourage the Expression of Feelings

It is both understandable and acceptable to cry at this time. Allow the client to speak about the personal effects of the situation.

### Address the Practical

Clients may be feeling overwhelmed by practical issues such as care for the animal, or financial issues. It may be necessary to address these issues first before owners can consider their emotional needs.

### Empower Clients to Actively Participate in Their Pet's Care

This includes enabling clients to make informed decisions. To make a difficult decision, people require information. It may be necessary to supply this information a number of times. The amount of information required will vary from client to client. The nurse with good communication skills should be able to ascertain whether a client feels well enough informed by asking appropriate questions and listening well to the responses. Clients will frequently ask for the nurse's opinion and will often use this to help inform their decision. This raises a number of issues. The cancer care team members have a considerable amount of power because they have both knowledge and experience. Therefore the opinion of the worker is likely to be valuable to the client. However, it is possible for this power to be used to sway or influence people from the course they were planning to take. It is therefore advisable to give an opinion only if well informed and in accordance with the rest of the team. The team that appears divided will cause a loss of confidence. If a client does not take the team's advice there will still be a need for support and a good working relationship.

### Privacy

Respect clients by allowing them to speak with clinicians away from other owners and staff. If possible an area should be set aside to allow people time on their own or, for families, time to speak with one another privately. If an owner is distressed, attempt to provide an alternative way out of the building rather than through the waiting area. Have respect for the fact that people may need time alone to reflect before making any decisions.

### Don't Assume You Know What Is Needed

Many factors will influence what an individual requires. Allow the client to guide you. What has suited one owner may not suit another.

### Spend Time with the Client

Introduce clients to other staff and familiarize them with the hospital. Get to know the animal and family and how the carers function, for example, do they make decisions as a unit or is one person usually responsible for decision making? Refer to the pet by name.

### Prepare the Client

Discuss the possible scenarios. If euthanasia is an option, describe what will happen and what the owner may see should he or she choose to be present (see also Chapter 14).

### Assess Support Needs

Most people will not ask for help or support. Owners may wish to avoid the stigma of admitting to distress. It is helpful if the nurse is able to identify this and offer support, even if it is not being requested.

### Reinforce Existing Support Networks

Encourage clients to enlist the support of family and friends or support from others, such as therapists or fellow members of a social club.

### Be an Advocate and Liaison

Owners may rely on the nurse to advocate for them and their pet if there are difficult issues to consider or problems with communication.

### Be a Resource and Facilitate Access to Information

Ensure that clients have verbal and written information and that they understand this information.

### Respect Spiritual Beliefs and Values

Ask owners about their beliefs. Phrases such as, "Fluffy is in heaven" can be either comforting or entirely inappropriate, depending upon a person's beliefs. People from diverse cultural backgrounds may have special needs.

### Do Not Make Promises You Can't Keep

Never assure an owner of an outcome. Phrases such as, "I assure you we will do everything in our power to help" can be reassuring without making guarantees or promises about the end result.

### Support Throughout the Journey

Although some stages in the cancer journey may be more difficult, such as diagnosis, terminating treatment, palliation, and euthanasia, owners may require support at any time. After death, support is increasingly considered the role of the veterinarian and support staff. Depending upon the constraints of the practice, it may be appropriate to send a card or flowers. In any case follow-up telephone support should be a part of good practice. If possible, the bill for services should be sent at a later date and not presented to the client at the time of bereavement.

## Societal Attitudes

The attitude of those surrounding an owner may impact on grieving. There can be a stigma surrounding the mourning for the loss or illness of an animal. Some people cannot understand the relationship the owner has had with a pet and cannot equate the loss of a pet with other losses. This is sometimes referred to as disenfranchised grief. By not acknowledging the grief over the loss of a loved animal, those surrounding a bereaved owner are contributing to the sense of devastation and causing the owner to feel isolated and alone. People may be told by well-meaning friends or relatives, "It's only a dog," "Thank goodness it wasn't one of your family members," or "You can always get another one." A support group in Pennsylvania catering specifically to bereaved pet owners identifies this social stigma as one of the main reasons people attend the group—they find they have no other venue in which they can speak about their loss. It is important that the health care team be mindful of this, as they may be the main or only point of support or validation for the grieving owner.

## Counseling

There are an increasing number of services providing therapy related to the loss of a pet. As a veterinary nurse or technician it would be useful to research the details and cost of those services in the local area. Services available will depend upon the size and population of the area. Providing a list of these counselors' names at the time of bereavement not only assists people to access support but provides validation that the grief is legitimate, whether or not they actually use the service. This should be raised sensitively; for example, the nurse could say, "You have had a lot happen in a short time. Some of our clients have found it helpful to have the names of people they can talk to." In larger urban areas there may be support groups for those who have suffered the loss of a pet. Many of these support groups are cofacilitated by a veterinary nurse and a health worker, such as a social worker or psychologist. The veterinary nurse is often able to recognize the need for such support, know whom to contact locally, and initiate this type of service.

## Special Considerations for Children

Children experience grief and their reactions are as varied as those of adults. Many workers are more concerned about speaking with children about death and dying than they are about speaking to adults. Societal attitudes have often dictated in the past that children must be protected from bad news. Many adults will recall being told, as a child, that their cat ran away or their dog went to live on a farm, only to realize as they grew older that the pet had died. Current thought suggests that keeping children in the dark can be emotionally damaging; children tend to be aware that something is happening but that it is being kept from them. They then imagine the worst possible outcome. They feel unsupported and betrayed when they eventually discover the truth. Parents or guardians should be allowed to decide how to approach a pet's cancer with their children. The nurse's role is to provide education and support during this process.

The age of the children will affect their understanding of the loss. Children up to the age of 4 years old do not understand the permanency of death and may believe the pet is going to return. They may exhibit some behavior changes such as clinginess or acting out in response to the loss. Children 5–10 years old are starting to understand that death is permanent. Children at this age often require a lot of information about what is happening. Adolescents generally have a similar understanding of death as adults do, but they may react more strongly, exhibiting signs of intense distress, social withdrawal, or mood swings. Children can be encouraged to be a part of the dying process with their pet. With issues such as viewing of the body and presence during procedures, the team should be guided by the parents and the child.

## Special Considerations for Elderly Pet Owners

Elderly pet owners have reported that the loss of a pet revives memories of past bereavements. It may also remind the elderly person of personal frailties and impending demise. Elderly owners are less likely than younger people, with children in the home, to get a new pet. For some elderly people the pet may have provided a sense of being needed. A pet also gives some stability and routine to daily activities. Some pets may signify a connection to a deceased partner, and the loss of the pet may cause memories of the loss of the partner to be relived.

## Other Pets

When an animal is sick or dies, the other animals in the home will be affected. They may search for the missing pet or wait for it to come back. The other pets in the home may behave differently or go off their food. Owners need to be made aware of this and be given some strategies to manage any behavior changes.

## Memorials

Some owners may be fearful of seeing a dead body. Others may wish to spend some time alone with their pet after it has died. Some may wish to have the veterinarian dispose of the body and others may wish to arrange for burial or cremation personally. A funeral or memorial of some type helps people to say goodbye to a pet, and it also allows them to acknowledge and celebrate the pet's life. Talking through the range of options available can be a helpful part of the grieving process. These may be varied and can include taking photographs and locks of fur, planting a tree on the burial site, writing a poem or song, having a plaque made, and conducting a service with family and friends. Although some requests may seem unusual, it is the role of the veterinary staff to assist with this wherever possible.

## Communication

The nurse-owner relationship can be quite significant over the lifetime of a pet, and particularly so at the end of life. The nurse must have an understanding of where the owner is in the grieving process and what he or she may be experiencing. This involves having difficult conversations about topics people usually prefer not to discuss, such as death and dying, or euthanasia. These conversations take place at a time when people are vulnerable, emotional, and being asked to make difficult decisions. It is therefore essential that the veterinary oncology staff communicate well with their clients. Good communication will lead to the provision of optimal patient care.

Owners enter a veterinary practice generally in a vulnerable or disadvantaged position. They are concerned for their pet, unfamiliar with the surroundings, and see the staff as experts. They may be afraid or embarrassed to ask questions. Owners may find it easier to talk to the nurse than the veterinarian. One of the most important components of a therapeutic nurse-owner relationship is trust. A nurse can gain the trust of an owner by employing a consistent and caring attitude, displaying competence and confidence with their pet, and being honest and open in all dealings. The nurse can take a collaborative approach to problem solving with the owner. A balance between maintaining professionalism and avoiding taking in an "expert" role is essential.

Good communication skills for nurses and technicians are important for many reasons:

1. Communication is an essential component of good practice.
2. Legal and ethical requirements require accurate documentation and consultation e.g., informed consent.
3. Owners require both information and support. This can be delivered most effectively through good communication with the health care team.
4. The health care team is most productive when its members communicate well with one another. Worker stress can be decreased, and mistakes or misunderstandings are less likely.

## Improving Communications

A number of strategies can be used to help improve communications with a pet owner:

1. Reflect on your attitudes and responses. Do you have a tendency to be dismissive, defensive, or overly familiar?
2. Try to put yourself in the client's shoes.
3. Provide information clearly. Avoid medical terms and jargon. Use clear everyday language.
4. Encourage questions.
5. Write down complex information, with diagrams if necessary.
6. Check understanding regularly.
7. Repeat and summarize. People may require information to be repeated a number of times, and on different visits.
8. Be mindful of language and cultural barriers.
9. Be mindful of physical barriers such as auditory or visual problems.
10. Encourage support persons to be present.

## Some Useful Communication Skills

### Empathy

"Empathy is the ability to accurately perceive another's emotions and communicate the meanings of feelings to the other through verbal and nonverbal behaviors" (Arnold and Boggs 1989). The nurse should be able to communicate an understanding of the owner's feelings without overidentifying. Some examples of empathic responses can be seen in Table 15.1.

### Active Listening

Listening is an essential communication skill. It is important to pay attention to what an owner is saying and to observe nonverbal cues as well. These may include pauses, lack of eye contact, and repetition of phrases. Each person who approaches a service is unique. A busy day can sometimes mean staff are unable to listen to each person individually. It

**Table 15.1.**  Examples of suboptimal and preferred responses to various client-communications situations

| Owner's Statement | Suboptimal Response | Why This Is Suboptimal | Preferred Response | Why This Is Preferred |
|---|---|---|---|---|
| "I'm sick of nobody telling me what's wrong with my dog." | "We are doing the best we can. We have a number of patients to see today." | Nonempathetic—creates barriers, lack of trust, and difficulty in building on relationship afterward | "It is difficult during this time of waiting for test results. It sounds like you are feeling a bit in the dark and frustrated. Perhaps we can ask the doctor to update you on the situation as it stands at the moment." | Acknowledges feelings, shows understanding, addresses practical issues |
| "I'm scared my cat will be in pain." | "We'll sort that out, don't worry about it." | Dismissive of fears, no real reassurance | "That is a very common fear, and I can certainly understand that your decision about treatment options will be affected by that. If you like, I can talk you through what is likely to cause the most discomfort for your cat and the pain relief that we may use." | Validates, acknowledges fear, and attempts to address |
| "No one knows how I feel about this dog." | "That's not true. We see people here with sick pets all the time. We understand how you feel." | Intrusive, assumes knowledge, denial of feeling | "It sounds like people around you aren't quite aware of how this is affecting you. Would you like to talk about your dog with us, or perhaps we can arrange some counseling or a support group for you?" | Acknowledges what was said, does not deny the statement |

is important not to make assumptions based on previous experience with a patient or what has happened in a similar case.

## Asking Open Questions

People can respond very differently to the same question, depending upon how the question is framed. For example, "You'd like to go ahead with the chemotherapy wouldn't you?" requires only a yes or no response. If the question were asked thus: "What are your feelings about treatment options?" a number of responses can be elicited. The original question would be answered, but the owner would also have the opportunity to talk through concerns about the treatment and ask further questions. A useful initial question to raise the issue of emotional support might be the following: "What has been the impact of this diagnosis on yourself and your family?"

### Avoiding Clichés

Statements such as "he's in a better place" or "it's only a dog/cat" should be avoided.

## The Communication Network

There may be numerous health professionals giving advice to an owner. Sometimes this information will be presented in slightly different ways. When the owner then repeats this information to other family members, he or she may present it differently again due to a lack of understanding, an omission of a piece of the information, or bias about the way they are feeling. It is not uncommon for people to end up with a very different interpretation from the original information given.

## When Communication Is Difficult

Maintaining good communication with clients is not always easy. Some people will be more difficult to work with than others. Some of the obstacles to good communication for veterinary technicians/nurses can include the following:

1. Workload, work stress, and time constraints can be daunting.
2. Emotionally challenging situations can be an obstacle; nurses may be afraid they will "make things worse."
3. Language or cultural differences can make communication challenging.
4. Owners with unrealistic expectations or very high needs, can become overwhelming.
5. Nurses might overidentify or find that a situation triggers an emotional response in them due to similarities in the case and the worker's own life. For example, a nurse may find it challenging to deal with a dying cat if the nurse's own cat recently died of the same disease.
6. Assumption by the worker that the owner will tell them how they are feeling may not prove true.
7. A team environment that doesn't encourage staff to communicate with clients can make supporting the client difficult.

Some of the barriers that may prevent owners from communicating with the cancer care team can include the following:

1. Not wanting to be a burden
2. A belief that nothing can be done
3. Not wanting to upset people
4. A fear of talking about dying
5. Social stigma
6. Not wanting to reveal weakness

### Managing Conflict in the Nurse-Owner Relationship

There are many reasons why owners may appear challenging or difficult in the veterinary cancer care setting. Owners who are demanding or have high needs can often be labeled

# What about the Nurse's Emotional Experience?

*Nicole Edwards*

A veterinary technician/nurse may be the individual clients turn to for guidance, consolation, and reassurance before, during, or after euthanasia of a pet because of their perception that the nurse was involved in the day-to-day care of the pet and is easier to approach than the veterinarian. Studies have shown that the health worker who is able to provide meaningful support and maintain good relationships actually has more job satisfaction.

## Working as Part of a Team

Nurses do not work with patients in isolation. They are part of a team consisting of veterinarians, other nurses and technicians, administration staff, and other support staff. They also liaise with a number of workers outside the practice such as pharmacists and nutritionists. It is vital that every team member understands his or her role in providing care to the patient and owner. The team must be united in focus and cohesive as a unit. In a multidisciplinary team roles must be established and negotiated. Given the difficult nature of the work, the team that does not act as a supportive unit will find there is a low retention rate, low morale, and disharmony, and inevitably the patients and owners will not receive the best care. A collaborative approach works best.

Nurses should familiarize themselves with the practice's policies and procedures. Regular team meetings and updates should be scheduled. Collaborative professional relationships ensure that a diversity of clinical skills are brought together to provide comprehensive cancer care.

Nursing staff members who experience a problem within their working environment should discuss it with their supervisor. This may involve a personality conflict or disagreement with a co-worker, stress related to workload, or a philosophical issue with the policies of the practice. The team should participate regularly in case discussion. An environment in which grievances can be aired should be encouraged. Team-building exercises or even professional assistance can be useful if needed.

## Conflict in a Team

This may be related to interpersonal difficulties, uncertainties about role delineation, differing opinions on managing care, or differing levels of experience and expertise within the team. Managing conflict within the team is not only the role of supervisors but of all staff. Open and ongoing communication is required. Both structured and unstructured discussions should be held regularly. The team should meet formally to discuss cases and issues within the practice. It is also useful for the team to communicate in less structured ways such as having lunch together or arranging social gatherings from time to time. A respectful atmosphere should be maintained by all. Workers should recognize common skills and negotiate roles. Above all, problems should be addressed as they arise, and not be allowed to develop into major concerns. If staff members are unable to come to a resolution on their own they may need to enlist the assistance of management or a professional mediation service.

## Ethical Considerations for the Nurse or Technician

The veterinary nurse will be faced with many ethical dilemmas during a career. Some of these issues are highlighted here in order that nurses may consider their own feelings or thoughts on these matters before facing them in daily practice.

### Working in Cancer Care

For those choosing to work in the cancer care field there are a number of ethical and moral considerations. There remain a number of myths surrounding the treatment of cancer, with many people still believing that a cancer diagnosis means death and that treatments for cancer are painful and intrusive. Any health professional wanting to work in this field should consider personal beliefs and feelings about cancer and its treatments.

### Benefits vs. Side Effects of Treatment

A question often arises: "Do the potential benefits to be gained from treatment outweigh the side effects?" If nurses have a clear understanding of the treatment regime and potential side effects they will best be able to advise and support pet owners.

### Cost of Treatment

Some owners cannot afford to have their animals treated. A common challenge for veterinary staff is finding a level of care that can help individual animals within the financial and time constraints of the family.

## Other Barriers to Treatment

Nurses may discover that owners have other barriers to accepting or accessing treatment: their own ill health, lack of access to transport, or other factors, such as an unsympathetic partner. Is it the role of the nurse to assist owners to overcome these barriers in order to provide the best care to a pet?

## Euthanasia

The procedure of euthanasia is discussed in detail in Chapter 14. Ethical considerations around euthanasia inevitably arise. Although the goal is always to allow the patient to die with dignity, comfort, and peace, any number of issues may present themselves to the technician/nurse at this difficult time. When is it the right time to euthanize? What if there is a difference of opinion about this? Nurses should bear in mind that many people will feel guilty if they decide to have their pet euthanized, and for some this will lead to complicated grief reactions.

# When You Disagree with a Pet Owner's Decision

One of the most difficult issues for a health professional can arise when clients do not heed medical advice. There will be occasions when the veterinary nurse disagrees with the care he or she is requested to provide for an animal. The nurse may, for example, feel that in his or her clinical judgment, an animal should be euthanized, but an owner may be insistent that further treatment be given. A nurse may feel that a pet is receiving inappropriate care, or insufficient attention is being paid to managing its symptoms. There are some strategies the nurse may find useful in these situations. Discussion of concerns with the veterinarian or supervisor is often a good starting point. It can also be useful to approach the client with concerns in a gentle and nonconfrontational manner. Perhaps the client is simply ill-informed or undecided about what to do. The nurse may also come to a better understanding as to why the client is taking a specific approach. Documentation of all concerns and discussions is essential. If the nurse feels overwhelmed by concerns and is unable to come to a resolution, it may be in the best interests of the patient and team if another nurse or technician is assigned to the patient. Finally, it may be helpful for nurses to remind themselves that they will not always hold the same values as others but that an open-minded approach is most productive.

# When Owners Are in Conflict

Nurses may find themselves dealing with pet owners who are in disagreement with each other over the care or treatment of their pet. A crisis such as a cancer diagnosis can intensify existing strengths and weaknesses in human relationships. The nurse needs to avoid taking sides and provide all parties with information and support. If necessary, it may be advisable to suggest professional counseling in order to resolve a serious disagreement.

## Maintaining Professional Boundaries

There will inevitably be some patients for whom nurses may feel a particular fondness or attachment. It is possible to act as an empathic and caring health professional and yet maintain a respectful professional distance. Familiarization with the practice's policies around professional boundaries and discussion with more experienced staff can help nurses in this area. Generally, for example, it is quite appropriate to show fondness for a patient by expressing sadness to the owner or providing comfort by way of a hug; however, it may not be appropriate to give the owner a personal telephone number so that the nurse may be contacted in off-duty time. Although it might be helpful to share private sadness at the time of a death it would not be appropriate to discuss at length personal experiences of loss and grief.

## Confidentiality

Again, it is important that the nurse or technician is familiar with the practice's policy on confidentiality. Clients have a right to privacy, and it is not appropriate to discuss a case outside of the confines of the practice or to identify a community member as a client. Clients may divulge sensitive information or act in a way that they would not want spoken of to others. As an example, in the veterinary cancer care setting it is vital to know that a client may be pregnant (see Chapter 8), even if they are not ready to share this information with family or friends.

## Documentation

Best practice dictates that accurate documentation is required in veterinary medicine. However, a dilemma arises when, as discussed, confidential or sensitive information is held. This information may require documentation, but it is important that all staff remember to respect the privacy of the medical record. In addition, value judgments, judgments about the client's mental status, or notes about the client's behavior should not be recorded unless genuinely necessary, and if so it should be done in absolutely professional terms.

## Complaints about Colleagues

As previously discussed, it is not uncommon for clients to manipulate staff or try to play one against the other. It is possible that the nurse or technician will be the recipient of a complaint about a colleague. Here, nurses face a dilemma. As advocates for their patients they are required to address any complaint whether legitimate or not, but as team members nurses offer collegial support and loyalty. This is an issue that needs to be handled with tact and sensitivity. The nurse should be familiar with the practice's complaint handling policy. Discuss with a trusted supervisor if this arises.

## When Your Own Issues Arise

Some patients will trigger emotional responses in a worker because they will identify with that patient or owner. The animal may look or act similarly to a beloved personal pet.

The owner may remind the worker of a parent or friend. This can come as a surprise to some workers who feel they are immune to such responses. If the nurse can acknowledge this response, management of this situation will be simpler and easier.

## Nurturing the Technician/Nurse

Veterinary nurses and technicians play an integral role in the cancer care team. They nurture and support patients, pet owners, and colleagues. It is therefore essential that some consideration be given to supporting and nurturing the nurse. Unfortunately, workers in caring professions often neglect their own emotional needs.

### Self Care for the Nurse

Technicians and nurses who understand themselves are in the best position to care for themselves. It is useful for nurses to reflect on their own personality, acknowledge strengths, and recognize limitations. A nurse should acknowledge that there will be times that this work is difficult or upsetting. Accept that it is reasonable to be distressed or frustrated on some occasions. When working in a demanding area such as oncology, the health professional who denies personal feelings will never be able to work as effectively as the person who recognizes and acknowledges emotion as a part of practice.

Some basic self-care techniques that should be incorporated into the technician/nurse's everyday life include the following:

1. Limit alcohol, particularly if being used to dull the senses or to help forget an upsetting incident.
2. Exercise regularly and maintain healthy eating habits.
3. Have an active social life outside of work. Spend time with family and friends. Enjoy hobbies and spending time outdoors.
4. Maintain healthy sleeping patterns.
5. Spend time with healthy animals and enjoy your own pets.
6. Indulge yourself occasionally. Have a massage, go out to dinner or take a trip.

### Stress, Compassion Fatigue, and Burnout

*Stress, compassion fatigue,* and *burnout* are words often associated with workers in caring professions. **Burnout** is the result of exposure to high levels of professional and personal stress without corresponding levels of support or resources to assist the individual to cope. People suffering from burnout may be irritable, insensitive, unmotivated, withdrawn, or cynical. They may feel overwhelmed by the challenges of their role but unable to address these challenges effectively. A poor working environment and doubts about ability to cope are usually significant contributors to burnout.

**Compassion fatigue** is different from burnout and is defined as the depletion of emotional resources that occurs as a natural consequence of caring for others. It is possible at any time in health workers' careers to feel some degree of stress related to work.

Another term often referred to in the literature is **vicarious trauma.** This occurs in workers who are exposed to highly emotion-charged situations and find that they are reliving the events and emotion of this time in the days or months afterward. This is commonly found in professionals such as paramedics or emergency department workers who are witnessing trauma frequently. However, it is possible that oncology professionals also will be exposed to particularly distressing or traumatic events that will continue to affect them for long periods of time. If a worker feels unable to stop thinking about an incident or is still feeling the emotion of it intensely after the event, or if sleep or normal routine is affected, it would be useful to seek professional assistance.

Technicians and nurses must remember it is normal to be affected emotionally when faced with an emotional situation. Repeated exposure to grief and loss can be confronting on many levels and a heightened sense of personal vulnerability is common. Working within professional constraints, high workloads, and team conflict can also be professionally and personally challenging.

Technicians can sometimes find it difficult to identify that they are suffering from stress. It is most useful to be aware of the signs of burnout and compassion fatigue before this occurs. Managers should also implement strategies to combat worker stress, because it is a major contributor to increased sick leave, high staff turnover. and low productivity.

Some strategies to combat workplace stress include the following:

1. Work on developing and nurturing a good team.
2. Set boundaries and know your limitations.
3. Develop good time management and organizational skills.
4. Work on collegiate relationships.
5. Access professional development and networking opportunities whenever possible.
6. Share resources.
7. Discuss problems with your supervisor and peers.
8. Remember the basic principles of self-care (above).
9. Access counseling if required.


## *The Role of Professional Counseling*

Seeing a professional counselor regularly or when the worker is feeling particularly in need can be invaluable in helping the oncology nurse deal with the stressors of this work. Counselors can also assist the nurse to find a balance between work and home life and provide an opportunity to debrief about work issues, discuss managing difficult situations, and negotiate team problems. Counseling can provide a venue for workers to express sadness and grief over the many losses with which they deal. Many oncology staff members report that counseling is an important part of their self-care.

In beginning a career in veterinary oncology, it is useful to remember that the technician/ nurse who approaches a pet and owner with compassion, respect, and understanding will make a positive impact on their lives. The nurse who remains open-minded and maintains a positive attitude will find a lot of satisfaction from working in this highly specialized field. Confidence and expertise will increase with experience. Above all, the best caregivers care for themselves first.

## Further Reading

Arnold E, Boggs K...
Nurses. Philadelph...
Dean K, et al. 2005...
...Work in Health...
Hodelmoser K, 2002...
...chosocial Ca...
...University P...

# Hematologic Emergencies

*Lee Garrod*

## Disseminated Intravascular Coagulation

Disseminated intravascular coagulation (DIC) is a state of hypercoagulation that can occur in cancer as well as other disease states. In this clinical syndrome, there is overstimulation with activation of the coagulation cascade. In many types of cancer there is upregulation of tissue factor (TF) and this results in factor VII activation, an interaction known to activate the coagulation cascade. What ensues is fibrin and thrombus formation (multiple small clots are formed in the microcirculation of major organs) with subsequent consumption of clotting factors and platelets. This consumption, together with fibrinolysis, which soon follows, results in bleeding. The body is, however, unable to respond appropriately to vascular or tissue injury because a stable clot cannot form. The hemorrhage associated with DIC can be subclinical to profound. The hypercoagulation and thrombosis causes organ damage from ischemia due to the impairment of blood flow and organ damage. The diffuse thrombosis leads to the morbidity and mortality of DIC.

Malignancy itself can directly cause DIC by a number of different mechanisms, including expression of tissue factor, procoagulation (activation of factor X), and hyperfibrinolysis. In addition, many patients on chemotherapy are immunosuppressed and are at risk of infection. Sepsis can result from immunodeficiency as a direct result of the malignancy itself or due to treatment and can progress to septic shock. These patients are at risk of DIC.

### Diagnosis

The presenting clinical signs and symptoms indicating DIC are potentially subtle, complex, and certainly not specific for this syndrome. Hemorrhage may be the only clinically apparent symptom, and yet it is the most advanced at this stage, which is why DIC is often a fatal syndrome. An underlying cause should be identified with this syndrome and DIC should not be assumed to be present just because of cancer (e.g., is sepsis also a possibility).

It is important to note there is no *one* test that is specific for DIC, and therefore tests must be interpreted with the clinical picture for an individual patient and the underlying disorder present. In suspected cases of DIC it is the trend of a test result, and not just a single value, that is best evaluated. A normal platelet count that remains normal and does not start to decrease would mean DIC is extremely unlikely. The D-dimer and FDP assay, when evaluated together, provide the most rapid and specific diagnosis of DIC. Ultrasonography of the liver and spleen in particular, with the use of an ultrasound machine with high-quality tissue Doppler capability, can be very useful in diagnosing the early thrombotic stage of DIC.

## Treatment

The treatment of DIC focuses on the priority of making the patient hemodynamically stable. This may include intravenous crystalloid, oxygen therapy, packed red blood cell or fresh whole blood transfusion, plasma transfusion, and/or antiarrhythmic therapy. Then, the underlying suspected cause of the DIC is addressed. Once a diagnosis of DIC has been established (or even if there is a high degree of suspicion that DIC is present), treatment should be instituted without delay. Unfortunately, there are no controlled clinical trials in veterinary medicine evaluating the effects of different treatments in dogs with DIC. Specific treatments for the DIC itself will depend on the stage (hypercoagulation vs. fibrinolysis and hemorrhage) at the time of presentation. Although heparin is the most widely used anticoagulant in the management of DIC, its use remains controversial because studies have not been able to conclusively demonstrate any improvement in survival related to DIC. Heparin is avoided in the face of moderate to severe thrombocytopenia.

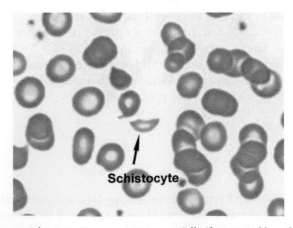

**Figure 17.1.** Schistocytes may be an indication of DIC, especially if supported by other findings.

## Summary: DIC

*Causes*

* Sepsis
* Malignancy
* Blood transfusions
* Liver failure
* Pancreatitis
* Immune-mediated disease
* Other causes

*Clinical Features*

* Client complaint
  * Asymptomatic
    * May be undetected until severe hemorrhage occurs
  * Dyspnea
    * Pulmonary thromboembolism (PTE)
  * Paralysis or limb weakness
  * Exercise intolerance
  * Bruising or bleeding
  * Mentation abnormalities
  * Gastrointestinal symptoms
  * Collapse
* Clinical findings
  * Symptoms and systemic evidence of DIC are based on the underlying pathophysiology of this process and may or may not include fever, hypoxia, acidosis, hypotension, and proteinuria. Depending on the severity of the symptoms of DIC, the patient may even demonstrate a clinical picture of shock.
  * Pulmonary dysfunction
    * From dyspnea to Acute Respiratory Distress Syndrome (ARDS)
  * Hypotension
  * Tachycardia
  * Hemorrhage
  * Jaundice
  * Gastrointestinal symptoms
  * Neurologic abnormalities
    * Localized intracranially
  * Cardiac arrhythmia

*Diagnostic Findings* (Note: there is no *one* test that is specific for DIC and therefore tests must be interpreted with the clinical picture for an individual patient.)

* Laboratory
  * Thrombocytopenia
    * Normal count excludes the possibility of DIC
  * Decreased fibrinogen

- Peripheral blood smear
  - Schistocytes = fragmented red blood cells (Figure 17.1)
- D-dimer assay elevated
- FDP (fibrin degradation product) assay elevated
- Anemia
  - Mild to severe depending upon stage of DIC
- APTT prolonged
- PT prolonged
- ATIII (antithrombin III) reduced
- Elevated liver values
- Elevated lipase and amylase
- Elevated renal values
- Acidosis
- Hypoxemia
- Hematuria or hemoglobinuria
- Bilirubinuria
- Positive blood culture
  - If due to sepsis
- Imaging
  - Radiography
    - Trace pleural fissure line (if PTE)
    - Pneumonia (if source for sepsis)
    - Intrapulmonary hemorrhage
  - Ultrasound
    - Pancreatitis
    - Abscess
    - Liver or splenic vascular compromise (vascular Doppler study)

*Management*

- Fluid therapy (crystalloids ± colloids)
- Oxygen therapy
- Low-dose heparin (use **WITH** blood products)
- Identify underlying cause
- Antibiotics
  - Specific for treatment of sepsis
  - For prevention of sepsis (bacterial translocation of the gut)
- Packed red blood cells or fresh whole blood
- Fresh frozen plasma
- Control overt hemorrhage
- Antiarrhythmic therapy

# Further Reading

Bick RL. 1996. Disseminated intravascular coagulation: objective and clinical laboratory diagnosis, treatment, and assessment of therapeutic response. *Semin Thromb Hemost* 22:69–88.

DeSancho MT, Rand JH. 2001. Bleeding and thrombotic complications in critically ill patients with cancer. *Crit Care Clin* 17:599–622.

Gordon SG, Mielicki WP. 1997. Cancer procoagulant: a factor X activator, tumor marker and growth factor from malignant tissue. *Blood Coagul Fibrinol* 8: 73–86.

Yu JL, et al. 2004. Oncogenes as regulators of tissue factor expression in cancer: implications of tumor angiogenesis and anti-cancer therapy. *Semin Thromb Hemost* 30:21–30.

Yu M, et al. 2000. Screening tests of disseminated intravascular coagulation: guidelines for rapid and specific laboratory diagnosis. *Crit Care Med* 28:1777–1780.

# Anemia

Anemia (meaning "without blood") is the deficiency of red blood cells (RBCs), hemoglobin and thus tissue oxygenation. Anemia is defined as a packed cell volume (PCV) less than 35%. A red blood cell or erythrocyte is produced by the bone marrow in response to stimulation by erythropoietin, which is produced in the kidneys. Hemoglobin is the oxygen-carrying molecule found within the red blood cell that transports oxygen from the lung to the tissue. The average life span of a red blood cell is 100 to 120 days in the dog and 70 to 78 days in the cat, much longer than the platelet (days) or neutrophil (hours). Anemia is the most common disorder of the blood overall. In cancer patients, a mild anemia is not uncommon. The anemia may be due to the cancer itself, anemia of chronic disease, immune-mediated destruction, hemorrhage, or long-term chemotherapy.

Anemia, in general, can be regenerative or nonregenerative. Regenerative anemia can be caused by excessive blood loss (acute or chronic hemorrhage) and excessive red blood cell destruction or hemolysis (immune-mediated destruction, blood parasites). Nonregenerative anemias are due to deficient red blood cell production or ineffective hematopoiesis. Causes of nonregenerative anemia include primary bone marrow disease or suppression, renal disease, nutritional deficiency (uncommon) and anemia of chronic disease. Anemia of chronic disease is the most common cause in small animals. This anemia is mediated by cytokines produced by inflammatory cells, which lead to decreases in iron availability, RBC survival, and the marrow's ability to regenerate. Treatment of the underlying disease results in resolution of the anemia. Primary bone marrow disease or bone marrow failure from any cause can lead to nonregenerative anemia and even pancytopenia. With diffuse marrow involvement, granulocytes are affected first, followed by platelets and then finally red blood cells.

Both cancer and its treatment can interfere with the supply of red blood cells by inhibiting production in the bone marrow. Most chemotherapy drugs can cause a degree of myelosuppression, and anemia is typically very mild if it does occur but may cause lethargy in the cancer patient. The most common hematologic effects from malignancy are anemia of chronic disease followed by blood loss anemia, microangiopathic anemia (a type of red cell destruction resulting in schistocytes in the peripheral blood commonly seen with hemangiosarcoma), and immune-mediated hemolytic anemia. In one study, cancer-related anemia, which is a common finding in dogs with lymphoma, was associated with a significantly decreased survival time compared with dogs without anemia.

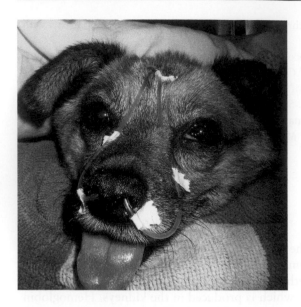

**Figure 17.2.** In a severely anemic patient nasal oxygen therapy may be indicated, in addition to red cell transfusion. When nasal oxygen is administered, the patient should be made as comfortable as possible to avoid unnecessary stress.

## Diagnosis

The clinical signs depend on the severity of the anemia and how quickly the anemia occurred. Patients that become anemic gradually have time to adjust to the decreased red blood cell count; animals that become anemic very quickly, however, may die because their bodies cannot compensate for the sudden loss in red blood cells and oxygen.

## Treatment

Treatment of the anemic patient focuses on the underlying cause in mild to moderate anemia. However, in cases where there is a life-threatening anemia, a blood transfusion may be necessary to stabilize the patient while the underlying cause is investigated.

## Summary: Anemia

*Causes*

❖ Decreased red blood cell production
- Anemia of chronic disease
  - ○ Any severe disease
- Renal disease
- Feline leukemia virus
- Bone marrow failure
- Nutrition
- Neoplasia
- Chemotherapy (usually mild)

- ❖ Increased red blood cell destruction (hemolysis)
  - Autoimmune disease
  - Red blood cell parasite
  - Toxin or chemical
  - Neoplasia
- ❖ Red blood cell loss
  - Bleeding from tumor
    - ○ Intestinal tract, spleen, liver, kidney, urinary bladder, others
  - Trauma or injury
  - Parasites (fleas, ticks, hookworms)
  - Coagulopathy

*Clinical Features*

- ❖ Client complaint
  - Asymptomatic (may be undetected unless moderate to severe hemoglobin decrease)
  - Lethargy
  - Depression
  - Weakness
  - Rapid breathing
  - Anorexia
  - Collapse
- ❖ Clinical findings
  - Weakness
  - Depression
  - Pale or icteric mucous membranes
  - Tachycardia
  - Heart murmur
  - Tachypnea
  - Organomegaly
    - ○ If due to a cancer process

*Diagnostic Findings*

- ❖ Laboratory
  - Anemia
    - ○ Decreased hematocrit or packed cell volume
    - ○ Normochromic, normocytic in anemia of chronic disease (ACD)
    - ○ Hypochromic, microcytic in blood loss anemia
  - Reduced hemoglobin
  - Peripheral blood smear
    - ○ Poikilocytosis (abnormal-shaped red blood cells)
      - ■ Schistocytes with hemolysis
      - ■ Spherocytes with IMHA
    - ○ Red blood cell parasites
    - ○ Presence of abnormal cells indicating cancer
  - Reticulocyte count
    - ○ Nonregenerative anemia = normal
    - ○ Regenerative anemia = increase

- Coombs test
  - Positive in 65% of cases with immune-mediated destruction
- Tickborne diseases titers
- Bone marrow aspirate
- Biochemical profile
- Urinalysis
- Fecal analysis
  - Parasites
  - Hematochezia
  - Melena
- Feline Leukemia (FeLV antigen) Test
- Imaging
  - Abdominal radiography
    - Possible neoplasm
  - Abdominal ultrasound
    - Organ abnormality may be apparent

*Management* (depends on the severity of the anemia and determining the underlying cause)

- Oxygen therapy (Figure 17.2)
- Identify underlying cause
- Control overt hemorrhage
- Packed red blood cell transfusion or fresh whole blood
- Erythropoeisis-stimulating agents (erythropoietin)
- Chemotherapy if cancer is the cause (e.g., leukemia)

## Further Reading

Barger AM, Grindem CB. 2000. Hematologic abnormalities associated with cancer chemotherapy. In: Feldman BF, Zinkl JG, Jain NL, eds, *Schalm's Veterinary Hematology*, 5th ed. Philadelphia, Lippincott Williams and Wilkens, 676–681.

Couto CG. 1990. Management of complications of cancer chemotherapy. *Vet Clin North Am Small Anim Pract* 20: 1037–1053.

Giger U. 2005. Regenerative anemias caused by blood loss or hemolysis. In: Ettinger SJ, Feldman EC, eds, *Textbook of Veterinary Internal Medicine*, 6th ed. St. Louis, Elsevier Saunders, 1886–1907.

Miller AG, Morley PS, Rao S, et al. 2009. Anemia associated with decreased survival time in dogs with lymphoma. *J Vet Intern Med* 23:116–122.

## Thrombocytopenia

Platelets or thrombocytes are produced in the bone marrow and are used to form blood clots and prevent bleeding. They survive in circulation for an average of 8 to 12 days.

When the number of platelets in the circulating blood falls below a normal range the condition is referred to as *thrombocytopenia*. Platelet production is specifically regulated by thrombopoietin, a hormone produced by the kidney and liver. Thrombopoietin deficiency is rare.

Thrombocytopenia, often defined as a platelet count below 200,000/µl is a common hematologic abnormality seen in oncology patients. Mild to moderate thrombocytopenia is a platelet count 20,000 to 200,000/µl and a severe thrombocytopenia is a platelet count <20,000 platelets/µl.

An abnormally low platelet count can arise from one or more of four general mechanisms:

1. Decreased platelet production (bone marrow disease/suppression, bone marrow infiltrative neoplasia, cytotoxic myelosuppression)
2. Increased platelet destruction or consumption (immune-mediated thrombocytopenia, disseminated intravascular coagulation)
3. Dilutional or distributional causes (fluid therapy or transfusion dilution, splenomegaly with sequestration)
4. Loss by hemorrhage (hemorrhage from tumor, clotting disorder)

Myelosuppressive drugs used in cancer chemotherapy can cause thrombocytopenia, depending on the dose and duration of therapy. Neoplasia of the bone marrow, while not as common as other forms of cancer in small animals, does occur and includes leukemias (many different types), lymphoma, myeloma, and mast cell neoplasia. Dogs and cats with bone marrow infiltration by a malignant process are more sensitive to the cytotoxic effects of chemotherapy agents that can result in thrombocytopenia.

Another possible mechanism of thrombocytopenia could be increased levels of inhibitory cytokines produced by or in response to the neoplasm. In one study, 10% of dogs with cancer had thrombocytopenia for a variety of reasons, but 61% of those had no identifiable cause. Dogs with hemangiosarcoma, lymphoma, and melanoma were at increased risk of developing thrombocytopenia. In another study 83% of dogs with cancer prior to chemotherapy had one or more coagulation abnormalities, 36% of which had thrombocytopenia.

Increased platelet destruction occurs as a result of immunologic causes, which are classified as immune-mediated (drug-induced, cancer, or without apparent cause) and infectious causes. Immune-mediated thrombocytopenia (IMT), also referred to as idiopathic thrombocytopenia purpura (ITP), occurs when the body's immune system destroys platelets. The diagnosis of immune-mediated thrombocytopenia lies in ruling out all other causes. Drugs including heparin and sulfonamides may be a trigger for immune-mediated platelet destruction.

There are many potential infectious causes of platelet destruction in which the reticuloendothelial system (spleen, liver, lymph nodes) takes the diseased cells out of circulation (e.g., Rickettsia, protozoa). In viral infection thrombocytopenia can be caused by myelosuppression (e.g., FeLV, canine distemper, rarely feline immunodeficiency virus[FIV]).

Increased platelet consumption occurs in patients with hemorrhage (from a mass or other coagulopathy) and in patients with disseminated intravascular coagulation. Disseminated intravascular coagulation (DIC) involves extensive intravascular clotting with dissemination of microthrombi consuming clotting factors, including platelets. DIC is discussed in detail earlier in this chapter.

In cancer patients undergoing chemotherapy, a degree of temporary thrombocytopenia may be expected and additional diagnostics may not be warranted. Therefore, knowledge of a cancer patient's recent chemotherapy history, including the drug, dose, and when the drug was administered, as well as the properties of the drug, is an important part of the evaluation.

## Diagnosis

Some animals with low platelets show no signs at all; others may be lethargic, anorexic, vomiting, or have bodily bruising and small hemorrhages in their mouth or nose. In cases of unexplained thrombocytopenia, additional diagnostics are necessary. When hemorrhage is present—as indicated by bruising (petechiation, ecchymoses), melena, or hematuria—the patient must be handled carefully while a full investigation of the cause of hemorrhage is undertaken.

Initial tests include complete blood count (CBC) with platelet count, blood chemistry, urinalysis, ocular examination, abdominal radiographs or ultrasonography, infectious disease titers, and coagulation profile. In evaluating the CBC, it is important that the laboratory technician manually read a blood slide when the blood machine reports thrombocytopenia, because platelets are sticky by nature and can clump together, resulting in a falsely decreased count. If the number is truly low, investigating the cause begins. Bone marrow evaluation is essential for differentiating hypoproliferative thrombocytopenia from increased destruction outside of the bone marrow where the megakaryocyte population in the bone marrow is normal or increased.

## Treatment

There is no specific treatment for thrombocytopenia. Rather, the treatment chosen, or whether treatment is indicated at all, depends on the presence and severity of hemorrhage. General precautions for thrombocytopenic patients include exercise restriction, minimizing venipuncture, avoiding intramuscular injection, and identifying and addressing underlying problems.

## Summary: Thrombocytopenia

*Causes*

❖ Decreased production
  ● Myelosuppressive chemotherapy drugs (usually temporary)
  ● Other drugs
    ○ Estrogen
    ○ Methimazole
  ● Bone marrow infiltration by malignancy
  ● Primary bone marrow failure

- Sepsis
- Viral infections
  - Feline leukemia virus
  - Feline immunodeficiency virus (rare)
  - Canine distemper virus
- ❖ Increased peripheral consumption or destruction
  - Sepsis (with or without DIC)
  - DIC (with or without sepsis)
  - Infectious
    - Rickettsia
    - Fungal (histoplasmosis, disseminated Candidiasis)
    - Protozoa (Babesia, Leishmania)
    - Nematode (heartworm)
  - Immune-mediated destruction (ITP)
  - Drugs
    - Sulfonamides
    - Heparin
- ❖ Altered distribution
  - Massive blood or blood product transfusion
  - Splenomegaly with sequestration
- ❖ Hemorrhage
  - Tumor bleeding internally
  - Coagulopathy with hemorrhage secondary to tumor, liver failure, anticoagulant rodenticide

*Clinical Features*

- ❖ Client complaint
  - Asymptomatic (may be undetected until severe hemorrhage occurs)
  - Bruising
  - Bleeding from any orifice
  - Exercise intolerance or collapse
  - Mentation abnormalities
- ❖ Clinical findings
  - No abnormal clinical abnormalities (especially if platelets are over 50,000/µl)
  - Ecchymoses or petechiae (if platelet count <50,000/µl)
  - Bleeding (if platelet count <25,000/µl)
    - Epistaxis
    - Bleeding from oral mucosa (gumline)
    - Excessive bleeding from venipuncture or catheter placement sites
    - Retinal hemorrhages
    - Hematemesis
    - Hematochezia
    - Melena
    - Hematuria
    - Hematoma (PT, APTT would be abnormal)
    - Hemothorax (bleeding tumor or abnormal PT, APTT)

- o   Hemoabdomen (bleeding tumor or abnormal PT, APTT)
- o   Hyphema
- Splenomegaly
- Evidence of thrombosis (results in platelet consumption)
  - o   Early disseminated intravascular coagulation (DIC)

*Diagnostic Findings*

- ❖   Laboratory
  - Thrombocytopenia
  - Peripheral blood smear evaluation confirms decreased platelet numbers
  - Anemia if bleeding
  - Coagulation screen
    - o   Prolonged PT, APTT, and low fibrinogen suggests DIC
  - Tick panel evaluation
  - FeLV/FIV testing
  - Bone marrow aspirate
    - o   Increased megakaryocytes = peripheral consumption or altered distribution
    - o   Decreased numbers = myelosuppression
    - o   Abnormal cells = bone marrow infiltrative neoplasia
- ❖   Imaging
  - Ultrasound
    - o   Bleeding abdominal mass (any organ)
    - o   Splenomegaly
    - o   Liver abnormality (coagulopathy)

*Management* (depends on the underlying cause and severity of bleeding, rather than the platelet count itself)

- ❖   Identify and treat the underlying disease
- ❖   Handle patients very carefully
- ❖   Avoid intramuscular injections
- ❖   Minimize catheter and phlebotomy sticks
- ❖   Stop any NSAIDs
- ❖   Delay myelosuppressive chemotherapy
- ❖   Control hemorrhage where possible
- ❖   Packed red blood cells or fresh whole blood if actively bleeding
  - *NOTE:* it is **NOT** feasible to transfuse platelets in dogs or cats in the majority of cases.
    - o   If life-threatening hemorrhage into the cardiopulmonary or CNS, platelet-rich plasma from fresh whole blood <12 hours old at room temperature only could be administered
- ❖   Epsilon aminocaproic acid (EACA) 250 mg/m$^2$ intravenous or orally QID for hemostasis in uncontrolled bleeding
  - Do **NOT** use if DIC suspected or confirmed
  - Do **NOT** use in cases of hematuria due to potential for urinary obstruction
- ❖   Chemotherapy indicated if infiltrative bone marrow neoplasia
- ❖   Immunosuppressive therapy indicated if immune-mediated thrombocytopenia (ITP)

# Further Reading

Grindem CB, et al. 1994. Thrombocytopenia associated with neoplasia in dogs. *J Vet Intern Med* 6:400–405.

Grindem CB. 2000. Infectious and immune-mediated thrombocytopenia. In: Bonagura JD, ed, *Current Veterinary Therapy XIII*. Philadelphia, W.B. Saunders, 438.

Madewell BR, et al. 1980. Coagulation abnormalities in dogs with neoplastic disease. *Thromb Haemost* 44:35–38.

Miller MD, Lunn KF. 2007. Diagnostic use of cytologic examination of bone marrow from dogs with thrombocytopenia: 58 cases (1994–2004). *J Am Vet Med Assoc* 231:1540–1544.

Ogilvie GK. 2005. Care beyond a cure: Oncologic Emergencies—Help!! *WSAVA Congress*, 542–545.

Reilly MP, et al. 2006. Prothrombotic factors enhance heparin-induced thrombocytopenia and thrombosis in vivo in a mouse model. *J Thromb Haemost* 4:2687–2694.

Scott MA. 2000. Immune-mediated thrombocytopenia. In: Feldman BF, Zinkl JG, Jain NC, Schalm OW, eds, *Schalm's Veterinary Hematology*. Ames, IA, Blackwell Publishing, 478–486.

Stockham SL, Scott MA. 2002. Bone marrow and lymph nodes. In: *Fundamentals of Veterinary Clinical Pathology*. Ames, IA, Blackwell Publishing, 228–252.

Sullivan PS, et al. 1992. Thrombocytopenia associated with administration of trimethoprim/sulfadiazine in a dog. *J Am Vet Med Assoc* 201:1741–1744.

# Neutropenia

Neutropenia is an oncologic emergency most commonly seen in cancer patients receiving myelosuppressive therapy. Neutropenia is discussed in detail in Chapters 13 ("Hematologic Support") and 18 ("Febrile Neutropenia").

# Febrile Neutropenia

## 18

*Lee Garrod*

Fever is defined as a sustained temperature in excess of 103 °F. Fever associated with cancer can generally be categorized into four major causal groups: infection, tumors (tumor-induced production of cytokines), allergic reactions to a drug, or allergic reaction to blood components in transfusion therapies. Fevers in cancer patients should be considered a result of infection until proven otherwise, because infection is a major cause of morbidity and mortality.

When a fever develops in a cancer patient, the individual must be thoroughly evaluated to determine the cause. A comprehensive physical examination should be performed and blood drawn for laboratory analysis.

Neutrophils are phagocytic white blood cells that defend the body against bacterial and fungal infections. When the neutrophil count drops too low, the body has difficulty fighting off infections. The neutrophil count is expected to drop below normal after treatment with many chemotherapy agents (transient myelosuppression), but it will typically return to normal quickly. This does not usually cause a problem unless the neutrophil count is below 1000/µl. The nadir (the lowest point the patient's cell count will reach) for neutrophils following a dose of myelosuppressive chemotherapy usually occurs approximately 7 days after treatment.

Neutropenic patients are immunocompromised and lack the ability to mount a full inflammatory response to infections. They are at risk of developing bacterial and fungal infections, with both pathogenic and opportunistic organisms, which are much more difficult to eradicate with appropriate antibiotic therapy. Therefore, fever may be addressed differently in the patient that has a normal neutrophil count than in one with a decreased neutrophil count.

Sepsis can occur in immunosuppressed cancer patients when there is severe or untreated bacteremia. Septic shock from overwhelming endotoxemia and sepsis causes circulatory collapse, which is often fatal as a result of the development of coagulopathy (DIC) and/or multiple organ failure.

## Diagnosis and Treatment

The degree and duration of neutropenia are the most important risk factors for developing fever after chemotherapy. Neutropenia and consequent infections usually occur approximately 1 week after a myelosuppressive chemotherapy drug is given; but for a few drugs the neutrophil nadir (and risk of infection) may be delayed or prolonged (see Chapters 8 and 13). If this happens, symptoms may include a fever, a poor appetite, lethargy, vomiting, and diarrhea. Typically, a complete blood count (CBC) is evaluated 7 days following a treatment. A rapid assessment of neutrophil numbers can be made from a fresh blood smear while the automated count is pending (Figure 18.1). If the neutrophil count is low and there is no fever, prophylactic antibiotics should be started to prevent an infection.

A patient with neutropenic fever is a true medical emergency, and timely administration of antibiotics can potentially prevent development of sepsis and death. A neutrophil count <1000/µl with a fever strongly suggests sepsis and mandates emergency management. It is imperative that the patient is hospitalized to administer antibiotics parenterally in order to rapidly attain therapeutic serum concentrations.

When a fever develops in a cancer patient, the patient must be thoroughly examined to determine the cause and source of infection if there is one. There are some situations in which the total white blood cell count can be normal or even high (e.g., leukemia) as a particular cell line is increased; but it is the absolute neutrophil count that should be paid particular attention to. The bacteria that are most commonly associated with infections in cancer patients arise from the dog and cat's own flora—often the gastrointestinal flora. A comprehensive physical examination should be performed and blood and urine submitted for laboratory analysis in order to identify the source of infection. Blood cultures may be helpful in neutropenic patients because they may provide a definitive diagnosis of the organism causing the infection and information about the sensitivity of the pathogen to antimicrobial agents. A negative blood culture, however, may result if the patient is not

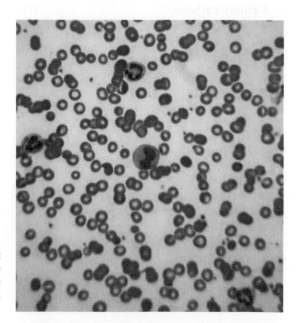

**Figure 18.1.** A fresh blood smear from a patient with normal numbers of neutrophils. Note the three neutrophils at the edges of this frame, and the monocyte in the center. (Courtesy of Dr. Dennis Meyer)

bacteremic at the time of the culture sample, there is insufficient blood, or the patient is on an antibiotic; and does not rule out sepsis.

Every patient that has a fever associated with myelosuppression should have blood and urine collected for culture before bactericidal antibiotic therapy is instituted. However, empirical antibiotic therapy should be commenced as soon as samples are collected, and while culture results are pending. Final antibiotic therapy is chosen based on culture of the offending organism from blood or urine and on identifying an antibiotic to which the organism is sensitive.

When a patient is severely neutropenic, the use of recombinant granulocyte colony stimulating factor (G-CSF: Neupogen) has not been found to be beneficial in cats and dogs with sepsis, presumably because these patients have high endogenous G-CSF.

## Summary: Febrile Neutropenia

*Causes*

* Tumors in the absence of infection
  * Release of cytokines by tumors that stimulate fever response
  * Tumor growth or spread into other tissues, including possible blockage
* Malignancy associated neutropenia or immunosuppression
* Chemotherapy-induced myelosuppression
* Blood component therapy reaction
* Drug allergy/anaphylaxis
* IV catheter, especially if neutropenic and long duration or aseptic (i.e. not sterile) placement
  * Neutropenia
  * Aseptic placement
  * Catheter duration
* Urinary catheter
  * Neutropenia
  * Aseptic placement
  * Catheter duration
* Multiple venipunctures
  * Especially if neutropenic
* Prolonged hospitalization
  * Nosocomial infection

*Clinical Features*

* Client complaint
  * Lethargy
  * Inappetence to anorexia
  * Diarrhea
  * Vomiting
* Clinical findings
  * Fever
  * Tachycardia
  * Dehydration

- Decreased blood pressure
- Diarrhea possible
- Abnormal lung sounds if pneumonia
- Heart murmur possible

## Diagnostic Findings

- ❖ Laboratory
  - May have low, normal, or increased white blood cell count. Attend to *absolute neutrophil count.*
  - Thrombocytopenia possible
  - Evidence of dehydration
    - ○ Increased total solids
    - ○ Increased hematocrit
    - ○ Increased BUN
  - Hyperglycemia
  - Hypoglycemia
  - Metabolic acidosis
  - Active urine sediment
    - ○ *NOTE:* in a neutropenic patient, pyuria may be absent.
  - Positive urine cultures
  - Positive blood culture
  - Positive catheter (intravenous) culture
  - Positive stool culture (if diarrhea)
  - Cytology of transtracheal wash demonstrates bacteria
  - Positive airway culture
- ❖ ECG
  - Sinus tachycardia
- ❖ Imaging
  - Radiography
    - ○ Possible pneumonia
      *NOTE:* may appear normal in neutropenic patient due to lack of neutrophil infiltrate
  - Echocardiogram
    - ○ Possible bacterial endocarditis
  - Abdominal ultrasonogram
    - ○ Possible pyelonephritis or other source

## Management

- ❖ Fever with normal neutrophil count, hydrated, no GI symptoms
  - Oral broad-spectrum antibiotic
- ❖ Fever with mild to moderate neutropenia (between 3000 and 1000/μl)
  - Restore adequate tissue perfusion if indicated by dehydration
  - Trimethoprim-sulfa
  - Fluoroquinolone
  - Amoxicillin or amoxicillin clavulanate
  - Delay chemotherapy

❖ Fever with marked to severe neutropenia (<1000/µl): assume sepsis
- Sterile IV catheter, isotonic crystalloids
- Fluoroquinolone plus cephalexin or amoxicillin clavulanate
- Dextrose if hypoglycemia
- Blood component therapy if indicated
- Delay myelosuppressive chemotherapy

## Further Reading

Abrams-Ogg AG, Kruth SA. 2000. Infections associated with neutropenia in the dog and cat, in Prescott JF, Baggott JD, Walker RD (eds): *Antimicrobial Therapy in Veterinary Practice*, 3rd ed. Ames, IA, Blackwell Publishing, 471–489.

Couto CG. 1990. Management of complications of cancer chemotherapy. *Vet Clin North Am Small Anim Pract* (4):1037–1053.

Moore AS. 2005. Practical chemotherapy. In: Ettinger SJ, Feldman EC, *Textbook of Veterinary Internal Medicine*, 6th ed. St. Louis, Elsevier Saunders, 713–720.

Zemann BI, Moore AS, Rand WM, et al. 1998. A combination chemotherapy protocol (VELCAP-L) for dogs with lymphoma. *J Vet Intern Med* 12:465–470.

# Metabolic Emergencies

Lee Garrod

## Hypercalcemia

Hypercalcemia is defined as a total serum calcium concentration greater than 12.0 mg/dl in dogs and greater than 11.0 mg/dl in cats or serum ionized calcium greater than 1.45 mmol/l (dog) and 1.38 mmol/l (cat). The ionized calcium is used to measure the body's biologically active calcium level. Calcium affects every organ system in the body and plays an important role in intracellular and extracellular metabolism, which controls many processes, such as nerve conduction, muscle contraction, coagulation, electrolyte and enzyme regulation, and hormone release. Calcium metabolism is controlled by hormones from the entry of calcium to the extracellular space from the bone and gastrointestinal tract to the excretion in the kidneys. Hypercalcemia can be the result of excess calcium entry into the extracellular fluid or of insufficient excretion.

Hypercalcemia is the most common paraneoplastic syndrome in cancer patients, and in turn, cancer is the most common cause of hypercalcemia in dogs and the second most common cause, next to renal failure, in cats. In cats with hypercalcemia, 30% have been found to have neoplasia; and up to 57% of dogs with hypercalcemia have been found to have neoplasia.

The malignancies most commonly associated with hypercalcemia include lymphoma, thymoma, anal sac gland adenocarcinoma, multiple myeloma, and pulmonary carcinoma in dogs and lymphoma and squamous cell carcinoma in cats. These cancers can result in hypercalcemia through one of three mechanisms: tumor production of a parathyroid hormone–related protein (PTH-rP and others), also referred to as humoral hypercalcemia of malignancy (HHM); local bone destruction (e.g., bone metastases) that results in release of cytokines (osteoclast activating factors); and tumor production of vitamin D analogues. Humoral hypercalcemia of malignancy is the most common mechanism that produces cancer-induced hypercalcemia. PTH-rP is very similar in structure to parathyroid hormone and therefore causes the same physiologic response as parathyroid hormone. The increased loss of calcium in the urine, decreased glomerular filtration rate, and increased tubular reabsorption lead to oliguria, further increasing the calcium.

Parathyroid adenoma (primary hyperparathyroidism) results in hypercalcemia by producing excessive parathyroid hormone. Parathyroid hormone causes increased release of calcium from bone by stimulation of osteoclasts, increases resorption of calcium from the distal tubules of kidneys, and increases calcium absorption from the intestines through activation of vitamin D.

Other causes of hypercalcemia in dogs and cats include acute and chronic renal failure, hypoadrenocorticism (Addison's disease), vitamin D toxicity (vitamin D–containing rat poison or topical ointments, or toxic plants), bone diseases associated with osteolysis, granulomatous disease (fungal) and idiopathic (cats only).

## Diagnosis

A high serum calcium level measurement should always be repeated to ensure that the result is not a laboratory error.

The symptoms of hypercalcemia are multiple and nonspecific, but they include depression, weakness, polyuria, polydypsia, nocturia, vomiting, and anorexia. The diagnosis can be made only by serum biochemistry. In-house serum chemistry analyzers and other instrumentation can measure the active (ionized) calcium or total serum calcium concentration. Total serum calcium includes the active (ionized) calcium and the protein (primarily albumin) bound calcium, in addition to other nonprotein calcium complexes. In dogs, alterations in the albumin and other plasma proteins can change this total calcium value. A corrected serum calcium in the face of hypoalbuminemia can be estimated by calculating: **Corrected calcium (mg/dl) = 3.5 − albumin (g/dl) + measured calcium (mg/dl)**. In cats, there is no linear relationship between serum total calcium and serum albumin and total protein concentrations. Whenever a calcium abnormality is suspected, ionized calcium is the best measurement to determine whether hypercalcemia actually exists.

Determining the cause of hypercalcemia can be difficult. The clinical signs are similar in patients regardless of the underlying cause and depend on the degree of elevation of the ionized calcium level. When faced with an elevated calcium concentration, it is important to ensure that it is not due to lipemia or hemolysis in sampling or laboratory error. An increase in the free ionized fraction of calcium can occur with acidosis. Cancer patients with acidosis therefore may have an increase in clinical signs of hypercalcemia. A thorough physical examination may detect abnormalities that may lead one to suspect a cause—for example, enlarged peripheral lymph nodes with lymphoma or perianal mass with anal sac carcinoma. The physical examination, however, may be unremarkable. Once an elevated serum calcium concentration has been determined to reflect true hypercalcemia, and the possibility of transient hemoconcentration (as in dehydration) has been eliminated, the patient undergoes further diagnostics.

## Treatment

The severity of the hypercalcemia and presence of dehydration will typically dictate the treatment plan for an individual patient. There are two objectives: reduce the elevated serum calcium level and treat the underlying cause. Symptoms are usually very mild in patients with a total serum calcium up to 14 mg/dl or ionized calcium up to 1.8 mmol/l. Symptoms are varied but more severe when the values are greater and serious renal damage can occur in addition to mineralization of soft tissues if the hypercalcemia is allowed to persist. Therefore, emergency treatment must be initiated with intravenous fluid therapy and sometimes specific drug treatment while the cause is being investigated. Severe hypercalcemia is usually associated with clinically evident hypovolemia, and the treatment plan must start with intravenous rehydration. Intravenous fluid diuresis with 0.9% sodium chloride (contains no calcium whereas lactated Ringer's does) helps enhance urinary excretion and prevent nephrotoxicity. Renal failure (calcium nephropathy) occurs if the calcium × phosphorus product exceeds 70. With fluid diuresis (two to three times maintenance rate), the potassium level must be monitored and supplemented if it decreases, especially in patients where there have been ongoing fluid losses or decreased intake. It is not necessary to get the calcium to within normal limits; a substantial reduction to minimize symptoms and secondary tissue mineralization consequences is often adequate. In cases of significant or persistent hypercalcemia, once the patient is well hydrated, furosemide can be used to promote calcium excretion. Prednisone, while helpful in promoting calcium excretion as well and reducing bone and intestinal calcium absorption, should not be considered until the cause of hypercalcemia has been established; this is because corticosteroids could mask lymphoma, making it difficult to diagnose.

## Summary: Hypercalcemia

*Causes*

❖ Malignant neoplasia (the following have been reported but there may be others)
  ● Lymphoma
  ● Leukemia
  ● Anal sac apocrine gland adenocarcinoma
  ● Thymoma
  ● Multiple myeloma
  ● Mammary carcinoma
  ● Pancreatic carcinoma
  ● Squamous cell carcinoma
  ● Nasal carcinoma
  ● Thyroid carcinoma
❖ Parathyroid hyperplasia, adenoma or adenocarcinoma
❖ Hypoadrenocorticism (Addison's disease)
❖ Renal disease
❖ Vitamin D toxicity
❖ Idiopathic (cats)
❖ Dehydration (mild hypercalcemia only)
❖ Lab error or interference
  ● Lipemia
  ● Hemolysis

- Mithramycin
  - If refractory to all other treatments
  - *CAUTION:* hepatotoxic and nephrotoxic

## Further Reading

Bergman PJ. 2001. Paraneoplastic syndromes. In: Withrow SJ, MacEwan EG, eds, *Small Animal Clinical Oncology*, 3rd ed. Philadelphia, W.B. Saunders, 35–53.

Elliott J, et al. 1991. Hypercalcemia in the dog: A study of 40 cases. *J Small Anim Pract* 32:564–570.

Feldman EC, Nelson RW. 2004. Hypercalcemia and primary hyperparathyroidism. In: Feldman EC, Nelson RW, eds, *Canine and Feline Endocrinology and Reproduction*, 3rd ed. Philadelphia, W.B. Saunders, 455–496.

Ikeda K, Ogata E. 1994. Humoral hypercalcemia of malignancy: Some enigmas on the clinical features. *J Cell Biochem* 57:384–391.

Kruger JM, et al. 2007. Hypercalcemia and renal failure. Etiology, pathophysiology, diagnosis, and treatment. *Vet Clin North Am Small Anim Pract* 26:1417–1445.

Midkiff AM, et al. 2000. Idiopathic hypercalcemia in cats. *J Vet Intern Med* 14:619–626.

Nelson RW. 2003. Electrolyte imbalances. In: Nelson RW, Couto CG, eds, *Small Animal Internal Medicine*, 3rd ed. St. Louis, Mosby, 828–846.

Savary KCM, Vaden SL. 2000. Hypercalcemia in cats: a retrospective study of 71 cases (1991–1997). *J Vet Intern Med* 14:184–189.

Schenck PA, et al. 2006. Disorders of calcium: Hypercalcemia and hypocalcemia. In: DiBartola SP, ed, *Fluid, Electrolyte, and Acid–Base Disorders in Small Animal Practice*, 3rd ed., Philadelphia, W.B. Saunders, 122–194.

Stewart AF. 2005. Hypercalcemia associated with cancer. *N Engl J Med* 352:373–379.

## Hypoglycemia

Hypoglycemia is defined as a serum blood glucose concentration of less than 70 mg/dl. Whether a patient is symptomatic depends on how quickly the blood glucose concentration decreases. Symptoms rarely occur until blood glucose is below 50 mg/dl. Glucose is the primary energy source of all cells, especially the brain. Glucose is also critical in lipid metabolism and the production of proteins, and it is the precursor for the synthesis of many substances, for example, glycogen.

Clinical symptoms usually reflect the rate of decrease of the blood glucose concentration, the underlying cause of hypoglycemia, and the chronicity of the problem.

Common causes of hypoglycemia include the following: insulin shock if the patient received insulin, adrenal insufficiency or hypoadrenocorticism (Addison's disease), liver failure, sepsis, xylitol ingestion, and neoplasia. Malignancy–associated hypoglycemia can be caused by a number of neoplasms, both pancreatic and nonpancreatic. The most common tumors associated with hypoglycemia are insulinoma, hepatoma, and carcinoma.

Insulinoma is an uncommon primary tumor of the insulin-secreting beta cells of the pancreatic islets and is a relatively common cause of hypoglycemia in older dogs. The majority of animals are middle age to older. Insulinoma is extremely rare in cats. The tumor produces increased serum insulin levels, and this in turn results in profound hypoglycemia, especially during periods of fasting.

There have been numerous extrapancreatic tumors associated with hypoglycemia, including hepatocellular carcinoma, leiomyosarcoma, hemangiosarcoma (liver and spleen), diffuse metastatic melanoma, and salivary gland adenocarcinoma. These tumors do not secrete insulin but instead are thought to cause hypoglycemia through unregulated production of insulinlike growth factors.

## Diagnosis

The majority of patients that present as an emergency with hypoglycemia have a cause other than cancer, and this is especially true in cats. In an emergency setting, an animal with diabetes mellitus that has received too much insulin for its blood sugar needs is the most common presenting cause of hypoglycemia. In nondiabetic dogs presenting with hypoglycemia, there are other considerations in addition to a possible cancer process. Physical exam findings are unremarkable in most patients presenting with a hypoglycemic crisis. The history of the patient—medications, including insulin, possible ingestion of xylitol—will certainly rule out these as potential causes. The signalment—young versus older—may also lead to a suspicion of one disease over than another (e.g., Addison's disease versus insulinoma).

Animals with insulin-secreting tumors of the pancreas may present with a history of episodes of weakness, ataxia, or incoordination, or seizure activity due to episodes of hypoglycemia. The history of symptoms is rarely acute. Neoplastic beta cells of the pancreas produce insulin, resulting in hyperinsulinemia. Excess insulin causes hypoglycemia, and this is the most consistent serum biochemical abnormality in animals with insulinoma. However, the serum blood glucose may actually be normal on initial presentation. If this is the case, the patient should be fasted and a serum glucose measurement repeated. Once the serum glucose decreases to below 60 mg/dl, a concurrent serum sample is collected to measure the serum insulin. In a normal animal, the insulin should be suppressed in the face of hypoglycemia. However, if it is normal or elevated, an insulinoma or insulin hormonelike-producing tumor should be suspected.

Additional diagnostic tests are likely needed to identify an insulinoma and exclude other causes of hypoglycemia. Insulinomas are not visible on radiographs of the abdomen, and pulmonary metastatic lesions are extremely rare. Ultrasonography of the pancreas can assist in identification of a nodule or mass, although the tumors are commonly very small (only 2 to 3 cm) at the time of diagnosis and can be difficult to detect. However, metastatic lesions in the liver or lymph nodes may be visible. The most common metastatic sites are the abdominal lymph nodes, liver, peripancreatic mesentery, and omentum. If ultrasonography is unremarkable and insulinoma still suspected, computed tomography (CT) or exploratory laparotomy may be necessary for definitive diagnosis.

## Treatment

Emergency treatment for a hypoglycemic crisis is symptomatic and is the same no matter what the underlying diagnosis. The goal is to alleviate clinical symptoms, not necessarily to have the blood glucose within normal range. Dextrose is administered with intravenous fluids until a patient is no longer critical, i.e., no longer seizuring.

Surgery is the primary treatment option for patients with hypoglycemia caused by a tumor. The postoperative prognosis and need for adjunctive care depends on the specific diagnosis and stage of disease; some have the potential to have fair to good outcomes.

For insulinoma, there is usually immediate and complete resolution of hypoglycemia immediately after surgical excision; surgery increases life expectancy over medical management alone, but it is rarely curative and in the majority of patients hypoglycemia eventually recurs. Postoperative complications such as pancreatitis may occur, but they are uncommon with proactive supportive care.

Medical management for hypoglycemia includes feeding frequent small meals, supplementing with glucocorticoids to counteract hyperinsulinemia, and limiting excitement and exercise. Prednisone increases hepatic gluconeogenesis and antagonizes the effects of insulin on peripheral tissues (insulin resistance); the effects may not be long-lasting, however, because the liver eventually maximizes gluconeogenesis and glucose release, and the peripheral effects of prednisone are eventually overcome. Diazoxide is an orally administered drug that can directly inhibit insulin secretion from beta cells and also stimulates the liver to produce more glucose resulting in increased serum glucose levels.

## Summary: Hypoglycemia

*Causes*

- ❖ Neoplasia
  - ● Insulin producing tumor (insulinoma)
  - ● Insulin hormonelike producing tumor
    - ○ Hepatoma
    - ○ Hepatocellular carcinoma
    - ○ Leiomyosarcoma
    - ○ Hemangiosarcoma
    - ○ Melanoma
    - ○ Adenocarcinoma
- ❖ Drug
  - ● Insulin
  - ● Xylitol
- ❖ Liver Dysfunction
  - ● Portosystemic shunt (PSS)
  - ● Cirrhosis
  - ● Acute liver failure
- ❖ Hypoadrenocorticism
  - ● Dog, rare in cat
- ❖ Sepsis
  - ● Overwhelming infection
- ❖ Decreased oral intake
  - ● Uncommon to cause decrease to point of seizures
- ❖ Laboratory error
  - ● Unseparated serum sits too long allowing the RBCs to metabolize glucose

*Clinical Features*

- ❖ Client complaint
  - Inappetence or anorexia
  - Polyphagia
  - Disorientation/incoordination
  - Extreme lethargy and weakness
  - Trembling or twitching
  - Seizures
- ❖ Clinical findings
  - Muscle weakness
  - Trembling or twitching
  - Tachycardia
  - Convulsions
  - Coma

*Diagnostic Findings*

- ❖ Laboratory
  - Hypoglycemia
  - Hypokalemia
    - ○ May be present in anorexic animals or diabetic patients
  - Elevated white blood cell count or profound neutropenia
    - ○ If overwhelming infection or sepsis
  - Bile acids abnormal
    - ○ If liver dysfunction or failure
  - ACTH stimulation test abnormal
    - ○ If hypoadrenocorticism (Addison's disease)
  - Insulin:glucose ratio >30
  - Insulin level normal or increased
    - ○ In the face of hypoglycemia, insulin dosing should be **DECREASED** in diabetic patients
    - ○ Rule out insulinoma or nonpancreatic tumor
- ❖ Imaging
  - Abdominal radiographs
    - ○ Not very helpful for insulinomas but extrapancreatic neoplasm may be apparent
  - Abdominal ultrasonography
    - ○ Evaluate the pancreas for presence of insulinoma and the liver and abdominal lymph nodes for local spread of the insulinoma
    - ○ Insulinoma may not be detectable if very small
  - CT scan
    - ○ May be the most sensitive imaging tool for insulinoma
  - Thoracic radiographs
    - ○ Extremely rare to see metastasis to lungs with insulinoma but other neoplasia possible

*Management*

❖ Emergency treatment of hypoglycemic crisis
  ● Intravenous crystalloid fluids to maintain hydration
  ● 1 to 5 ml 50% dextrose slow intravenously over 10 minutes
❖ Medications
  ● Prednisone
    ○ 0.5 to 2 mg/kg PO divided BID
    ○ Beneficial effects may wear off quickly
  ● Diazoxide
    ○ 10 to 40 mg/kg divided BID
    ○ Adverse effect: sodium retention
    ○ Hydrochlorothiazide can be added to counteract the adverse effects secondary to this medication
  ● Octreotide
❖ Diet
  ● High fat, high protein and low carbohydrates (carbohydrates cause insulin surges) or at least complex carbohydrates if present (oatmeal, bran, brown rice)
  ● Frequent small meals: 3 to 6 times a day
❖ Manage the underlying cause
❖ Surgery and/or chemotherapy

# Further Reading

Cohen M, et al. 2003. Gastrointestinal leiomyosarcoma in 14 dogs. *J Vet Intern Med* 17:107–110.

Feldman EC, Nelson RW. 2004. Beta-cell neoplasia: insulinoma. In: Feldman EC, Nelson RW, eds, *Canine and Feline Endocrinology and Reproduction*, 3rd ed. Philadelphia, W.B. Saunders, 642–643.

Fischer JR, et al. 2000. Glucagon constant-rate infusion: a novel strategy for the management of hyperinsulinemic-hypoglycemic crisis in the dog. *J Am Anim Hosp Assoc* 36:27–32.

Leifer CE, et al. 1985. Hypoglycemia associated with nonislet cell tumor in 13 dogs. *J Am Vet Med Assoc* 186:53–55.

Simpson KW, et al. 1995. Evaluation of the long-acting somatostatin analogue octreotide in the management of insulinoma in three dogs. *J Small Anim Pract* 36:161–165.

Tobin RL, et al. 1999. Outcome of surgical versus medical treatment of dogs with beta cell neoplasia: 39 cases (1990–1997). *J Am Vet Med Assoc* 215:226–230.

# Hypokalemia

Normal plasma potassium [$K^+$] is 3.5–5.0 mmol/l. Symptomatic hypokalemia usually occurs with a plasma potassium [$K^+$] <2.5 mmol/l. Potassium is important to maintain heart, gastrointestinal, and neuromuscular function through establishing and maintaining resting membrane potentials. The body's potassium stores are maintained by food ingestion and must keep up with potassium normally lost in the urine. When intake decreases and excretion increases, hypokalemia is the consequence. Hypomagnesemia can lead to potassium depletion and hypokalemia because it reduces intracellular potassium movement and also leads to decreased renal potassium resorption in the loop of Henle and the cortical collecting duct.

Hypokalemia can cause profound muscle weakness. Although cancer patients rarely present as an emergency due to acute hypokalemia unless profoundly cachexic, it is worth noting in this section because various severities of hypokalemia are associated with problems encountered commonly in cancer patients. The presence of concurrent hypokalemia in these patients may exacerbate their symptoms.

Although renal failure is by far the most common cause of hypokalemia in dogs and cats, especially through loss of potassium in urine, potassium can also be lost excessively through the gastrointestinal tract. Therefore, decreased intake may deplete the body's potassium stores, as seen with the anorexic patient. Anorexia can result from the cancer itself, or secondary to chemotherapy. Vomiting and diarrhea may disrupt electrolyte homeostasis, resulting in hypokalemia. Metabolic alkalosis secondary to vomiting will increase mobilization of potassium from the extracellular space to the intracellular space. Acute renal failure caused by cancer or nephrotoxic drugs can also result in hypokalemia. However, adequate hydration and diuresis in patients receiving a nephrotoxic drug minimizes the occurrence of the latter.

## Diagnosis

The hypokalemic patient will present with symptoms of their primary disease and, depending on the degree of hypokalemia, will have mild lethargy to profound weakness. In the author's opinion, cats will more commonly suffer the clinical consequences of hypokalemia. Mild hypokalemia (3.0 to 3.5 mmol/l) will rarely result in clinical symptoms. Neuromuscular weakness, gastrointestinal disturbance, and cardiac abnormalities can be prominent when the potassium is below 2.5 mmol/l. Both hypokalemia and hyperkalemia can be arrhythmogenic. Hypokalemia predisposes the myocardium to after-depolarizations and can result in ectopic beats. Hypokalemia can cause a metabolic alkalosis, which can worsen potassium imbalance because alkalosis can prolong hypokalemia.

## Treatment

Therapy for hypokalemia is directed at correcting the underlying cause (loss) and starting replacement with a potassium salt (potassium chloride, potassium phosphate). Patients with severe or acute hypokalemia are initially treated with intravenous potassium chloride (KCl) solution in 0.9% NaCl. Patients with severe hypokalemia should be potassium "loaded" but the rate of potassium chloride supplementation **should not exceed 0.5 mEq/ kg/hr**. The excessive amounts of potassium lost through the urinary and gastrointestinal tracts, even if only mild, can worsen in patients on intravenous fluids through dilution, and supplementation is necessary in these patients as well.

## Summary: Hypokalemia

### Causes

* ❖ Decreased intake
  * Anorexia due to cancer
  * Anorexia due to chemotherapy
* ❖ Increased gastrointestinal losses
  * Vomiting
  * Diarrhea
* ❖ Renal failure
  * Polyuric chronic renal failure
  * Acute tubular necrosis
* ❖ Metabolic alkalosis
  * Increased mobilization of [$K^+$] into cells (vomiting)
* ❖ Drugs
  * Diuretics
  * Nephrotoxic drugs

### Clinical Features

* ❖ Client complaint
  * Inappetence or anorexia
  * Vomiting
  * Diarrhea
  * Constipation
  * Polyuria
  * Extreme lethargy and weakness
* ❖ Clinical findings
  * Muscle weakness
  * Dehydration
  * Tachycardia
  * Arrhythmias

### Diagnostic Findings

* ❖ Laboratory
  * Hypokalemia
  * Hypomagnesemia
  * Metabolic acidosis
  * Metabolic alkalosis
  * Elevated renal values
    * ○ Polyuric renal failure
    * ○ Acute tubular damage
* ❖ ECG
  * Elevated P wave
  * Flattened T wave
  * Increased R wave amplitude

- S-T segment depression
- Prolongation of the QT interval

*Management*

- ❖ Treat the underlying cause if possible (e.g., vomiting)
- ❖ Intravenous crystalloid fluid therapy
  - Correct hydration
  - Caution to monitor further potassium dilution
- ❖ Potassium supplementation
  - Oral potassium solution if very mild
  - Mild hypokalemia (serum $K^+$ = 3.0–3.5 mmol/l): 2–3 mEq KCl/kg
  - Moderate hypokalemia (serum $K^+$ = 2.5–3.0 mmol/l): 3–5 mEq KCl/kg
  - Severe hypokalemia (serum $K^+$ = <2.5 mmol/l): 5–10 mEq KCl/kg
  - Do not exceed 0.5 mEq/kg/hr

# Further Reading

Church D. 2005. Electrolyte disorders. In: Ettinger SJ, Feldman EC, eds, *Textbook of Veterinary Internal Medicine*, 6th ed. St. Louis, Elsevier Saunders, 236–240.

Feldman EC, Ettinger SJ. 1977. Electrocardiographic changes associated with electrolyte disturbances. *Vet Clin North Am Small Anim Pract* 7:487–496.

Phillips SL, Polzin DJ. 1998. Clinical disorders of potassium homeostasis. Hyperkalemia and hypokalemia. *Vet Clin North Am Small Anim Pract* 2:545–566.

# Hypomagnesemia

The normal range for serum magnesium [Mg] in the dog is 1.7 to 2.4 mg/dl and 1.8 to 2.5 mg/dl in the cat. Hypomagnesemia occurs when the serum ionized magnesium is less than 1.2 mg/dl. Although only less than 1% of the body's total magnesium is in the plasma, magnesium is an essential mineral and is a cofactor to multiple enzyme reactions in the body, most importantly forming and using ATP. Magnesium is an important regulator of sodium, potassium, and calcium channels. In addition, magnesium causes bronchodilation through relaxation of bronchial smooth muscle and has many neurologic effects such as reducing electrical excitation and blocking acetylcholine.

## Diagnosis

Hypomagnesemia is included in this textbook because, in addition to hypokalemia, it can be associated with generalized muscle weakness when mild. Hypomagnesemia causes cells to lose potassium that is subsequently excreted by the kidneys, resulting in hypokalemia. In more severe hypomagnesemia, clinical symptoms are similar to symptoms seen with hypocalcemia (depression, ataxia, agitation, tremors, seizures). In humans, the development of hypomagnesemia during an ICU stay is associated with a worse prognosis. If a patient is diagnosed with hypokalemia or hypocalcemia and is not responding to treatment, it may be associated with hypomagnesemia, and thus it is important to measure this cation.

## Treatment

Life-threatening hypomagnesemia with severe clinical signs (ventricular arrhythmias) can be treated with magnesium sulfate 50% or magnesium chloride 50% administered intravenously slowly. Less severe deficiencies are treated with a constant rate infusion with magnesium sulfate 50% or magnesium chloride diluted to less than 20% in 5% dextrose in water.

## Summary: Hypomagnesemia

*Causes*

❖ Decreased intake
 ● Anorexia due to cancer
 ● Anorexia due to chemotherapy
❖ Increased gastrointestinal losses
 ● Vomiting
 ● Diarrhea
❖ Renal failure
 ● Polyuric chronic renal failure
 ● Acute tubular necrosis
❖ Metabolic alkalosis
❖ Drugs
 ● Diuretics
 ● Nephrotoxic chemotherapy drugs
  ○ Cisplatin (profound)
  ○ Doxorubicin (in cats)
  ○ Methotrexate
  ○ Streptozotocin

*Clinical Features*

❖ Client complaint
 ● Anorexia
 ● Nausea/vomiting
 ● Diarrhea
 ● Depression
 ● Extreme lethargy and weakness
 ● Incoordination
 ● Ataxia
 ● Tremors
 ● Seizures

❖ Clinical findings
  ● Muscle weakness
  ● Dehydration
  ● Tachycardia
  ● Arrhythmias
    ○ Ventricular arrhythmias
  ● Tremors
  ● Seizures

*Diagnostic Findings*

❖ Laboratory
  ● Hypomagnesemia
  ● Hypokalemia
  ● Hypocalcemia
  ● Metabolic acidosis
  ● Metabolic alkalosis
  ● Elevated renal values
    ○ Polyuric renal failure
    ○ Acute tubular damage
❖ ECG
  ● Elevated P wave
  ● Flattened T wave
  ● Increased R wave amplitude
  ● S-T segment depression
  ● Prolongation of the QT interval

*Management*

❖ Eliminate the underlying cause if possible
❖ Intravenous crystalloid fluid therapy
  ● Correct hydration
❖ Magnesium chloride 50% or magnesium sulfate 50% supplementation
  ● Mg < 1.2 mg/dl
    ○ 0.75 to 1.0 mEq/kg/day
    ○ Administer in dextrose in water as CRI

# Further Reading

Dhupa N, Proulx J. 1998. Hypocalcemia and hypomagnesemia. *Vet Clin North Am Small Anim Pract* 28:587–608.

Schonwald S. 2004. Magnesium. In: Dart RC, ed, *Medical Toxicology*, 3rd ed. Philadelphia, Lippincott Williams and Wilkins, 901–902

Soliman HM, et al. 2003. Development of ionized hypomagnesemia is associated with higher mortality rates. *Crit Care Med* 31:1082–1087.

## Tumor Lysis Syndrome

Tumor lysis syndrome (TLS) involves several potentially life-threatening electrolyte metabolic derangements including hyperkalemia, hyperphosphatemia, and secondary hypocalcemia. TLS results from treatment-related cell lysis (apoptosis) and can occur after chemotherapy or radiotherapy (usually after the initial treatment). This syndrome is rarely encountered in veterinary medicine, but when it does occur it is most commonly seen within 48 hours following initial chemotherapy of large-volume, highly chemosensitive tumors with a high proliferation rate, such as high-grade lymphoma with a large tumor burden or acute lymphoblastic leukemia. Therefore, an index of suspicion should be maintained when evaluating the patient who has undergone recent chemotherapy.

In TLS, the massive release of intracellular tumor products and metabolites after tumor cell death can lead to acute renal failure. The volume of products from the damaged cells overwhelms the body's ability to eliminate them. Intracellular potassium is released from the tumor cells which further decreases renal function and leads to hyperkalemia. Rapidly dividing tumor cells contain an increased amount of phosphorus relative to the normal cell (4× the amount). Phosphorus increases and can result in profound hypocalcemia as the phosphorus binds with the calcium.

### Diagnosis

The symptoms of TLS are usually nonspecific, but they range from vomiting to collapse. The presenting symptoms may indicate dehydration only or uremia and volume overload. Severe cases can present with seizures or weakness or collapse secondary to cardiac arrhythmias. Hyperkalemia produces life-threatening cardiac arrhythmias. Hyperphosphatemia is manifested as neurologic symptoms (including seizures) and arrhythmias. Once the calcium × phosphorus product exceeds 70, nephrocalcinosis occurs, resulting in renal failure. Other products are also released that damage the tubules of the kidneys. The renal failure worsens in the face of hypovolemia or dehydration.

The diagnosis is made through laboratory evaluation of multiple parameters and the recent history of starting chemotherapy or radiotherapy. Laboratory values often show elevated renal parameters, elevated potassium, elevated phosphorus, and a decreased calcium level. The electrocardiogram abnormalities will be the result of the severity of the electrolyte abnormalities (especially potassium) and a severe bradycardia is evident with significant hyperkalemia.

### Treatment

TLS is a serious emergency if it occurs, not only because of the severity of the electrolyte disturbances seen, but because of the multiple electrolyte abnormalities that occur at once. Patients require immediate hospitalization for treatment and cardiac monitoring. Intravenous fluids are administered to preserve renal function, but caution must be used in the face of cardiac abnormalities to avoid volume overload. Hyperkalemia is treated aggressively with the medications outlined in Table 19.1. Similarly, hypocalcemia is treated if the patient is symptomatic.

## Summary: Tumor Lysis Syndrome

*Causes*

- ❖ Neoplasia
  - ● Lymphoma
    - ○ Dog and cat reported
  - ● Leukemia, particular ALL (acute lymphoblastic leukemia)
- ❖ Recent chemotherapy or radiotherapy
  - ● Predisposed if preexisting renal disease
  - ● Large tumor or highly proliferative neoplasia

*Clinical Features*

- ● Weakness
- ● Vomiting
- ● Diarrhea
- ● Bradycardia
- ● Collapse
- ● Death

*Diagnostic Findings*

- ❖ Laboratory
  - ● Hyperkalemia
  - ● Hyperphosphatemia
  - ● Hypocalcemia
  - ● Elevated renal values (BUN and creatinine)
- ❖ Imaging
  - ● None indicated, although massive decrease in previously identified tumor burden would increase suspicion for TLS
- ❖ ECG
  - ● Bradycardia
  - ● Diminished P wave amplitude
  - ● Increased PR interval
  - ● Increased QRS interval

*Management*

- ❖ Intravenous fluid therapy with 0.9% sodium chloride for diuresis
- ❖ Emergency treatment of hyperkalemia if ECG abnormalities
  - ● 1 to 2 mEq /kg sodium bicarbonate IV slow, or
  - ● 1 to 2 ml/kg 50% dextrose IV slow, or
  - ● 0.5 to 1 U/kg regular insulin IV WITH 2 g 50% dextrose per unit insulin, or
  - ● 0.5 to 1 ml/kg of 10% calcium gluconate IV slow over 15 minutes closely monitoring the electrocardiogram monitor

**Table 19.1.** Treatment of metabolic abnormalities

| Problem | Intervention | Dosages | Comments |
|---|---|---|---|
| Hypercalcemia | Intravenous 0.9% NaCl | 2 to 3 times maintenance after rehydration | |
| | Furosemide | 1–4 mg/kg SID to TID orally **OR** 1–5 mg/kg/hr with diuresis titrating to effect | ONLY if well hydrated |
| | Prednisone **OR** | 1 mg/kg/BID | Prednisone or dexamethasone may interfere with accurate diagnosis if done before confirmed |
| | Dexamethasone | 0.1–0.2 mg/kg SC or IV every 12 hr | |
| | Pamidronate **OR** | 0.65–2.0 mg/kg intravenous **OR** 1.3 mg/kg in 150 ml saline intravenously over 2 hr | Safe Effective Expensive Use if severe and diuresis and furosemide ineffective or severe hypercalcemia Can repeat in 1–3 weeks |
| | Etidronate | 5 mg/kg daily orally | |
| | Calcitonin | (dog) 4.5–8 IU/kg SC every 8 hr **OR** 5 IU/kg SC every 12 hr (cat) 4 IU/kg IM every 12 hr | Expensive Short-lived efficacy |
| Hypoglycemia | Karo syrup | 0.5–1 ml/kg orally | Only if conscious and alert |
| | Dextrose 50% IV | 1–5 ml of 50% dextrose intravenously over 10–15 min IV crystalloids with 2.5–5% dextrose over 24–48 hr | Avoid excess as can cause rebound hypoglycemia |
| | Prednisone | 0.25–0.5 mg/kg orally every 12 hr: dose may be increased up to 2–3 mg/kg every 12 hr | Adverse effects may be uncomfortable for owners at higher doses |
| | Diazoxide | Initial dose 5 mg/kg orally every 12 hr Titrate upward to 30 mg/kg every 12 hr if needed | Used in conjunction with prednisone |
| | Glucagon | 5 ng/kg/min intravenous constant rate infusion; can titrate up to 30 ng/kg/min | Reconstitute 1 mg and add to 1 liter 0.9% NaCl for a 1 µg/ml concentration to make the CRI rate reasonable |
| | Octreotide | 20–40 µg SC every 12 hr; increase to every 8 hr if needed | Expensive Safe May be ineffective in many Use as last resort |

**Table 19.1.** *Continued*

| Problem | Intervention | Dosages | Comments |
|---|---|---|---|
| Hypokalemia | Mild (3.0–3.5 mmol/l) | Oral potassium supplementation if hydration adequate; otherwise, 2–3 mEq KCl/kg in crystalloid fluid intravenously | IV solutions: Do not exceed 0.5 mEq/kg/hour |
| | Moderate (2.5–3.0 mmol/l) | 3–5 mEq KCl/kg in crystalloid fluid intravenously | |
| | Severe (less than 2.5 mmol/l) | 5–10 mEq KCl/kg in crystalloid fluid intravenously | |
| Hypomagnesemia | Mild to moderate (<1.2 mg/dl) | Magnesium sulfate 50% **OR** magnesium chloride 10% in 5% dextrose in water at 0.75–1.0 mEq/kg/d CRI | |
| | Severe (life-threatening) | Magnesium sulfate 50% **OR** magnesium chloride 10% at 0.15–0.3 mEq/kg intravenously slow over 15 min | |
| Hyperphosphatemia | Minimize phosphate intake Phosphorus binders (aluminum hydroxide) | Aluminum hydroxide 500 mg with food every 12–24 hr | Phosphate binders may interfere with drug absorption |
| Hyperkalemia | Regular insulin | 0.5–1 IU/kg IV | Give WITH 2 g 50% dextrose per unit insulin |
| | Dextrose 50% intravenous | 1–2 ml/kg intravenously | Give slowly IV |
| | Calcium gluconate 10% intravenous | 0.5–1 ml/kg intravenously | Do not give with bicarbonate; monitor ECG with administration; can be repeated as needed |
| | Sodium bicarbonate | 1–2 mEq/kg intravenously | Use if acidosis Give slowly IV |
| Hypocalcemia | Calcium gluconate 10% intravenous | 0.5–1.5 ml/kg of 10% calcium gluconate **OR** 5–15 mg/kg/hr of 10% calcium gluconate IV CRI | Use only if symptomatic; caution if severe hyperphosphatemia Continuous electrocardiogram monitoring necessary |

## Further Reading

Calia CM, et al. 1996. Acute tumor lysis syndrome in a cat with lymphoma. *J Vet Intern Med* 10:409–411.

Couto CG. 1990. Management of complications of cancer chemotherapy. *Vet Clin North Am Small Anim Pract* 20:1037–1050.

Lanig EJ, Carter RF. 1988. Acute tumor lysis syndrome following treatment of canine lymphoma. *J Am Anim Hosp Assoc* 24:691–696.

# 20 Anaphylaxis

*Lee Garrod*

An allergic reaction can occur when the body reacts negatively to a foreign substance (antigen) and triggers the immune system. The immune system overreacts, resulting in a hypersensitivity or allergic reaction. Anaphylaxis is a severe allergic reaction to a foreign agent that affects the entire body and can be fatal. Anaphylactic reactions to some chemotherapy drugs may occur within seconds or minutes if given intravenously.

There are 2 types of anaphylaxis: anaphylactic reaction and anaphylactoid reaction. The clinical picture of an anaphylactic and anaphylactoid reaction does not differ.

In an anaphylactic reaction, the immune system has become sensitized to an antigen to which it has been previously exposed (e.g., a drug), thus forming antibodies (IgE) such that on subsequent exposure, they trigger a sudden, severe systemic allergic reaction through the release of histamine and other vasoactive substances (leukotrienes, prostaglandins, heparin) from basophils (bloodstream) and mast cells (tissue).

An anaphylactoid reaction also results in the immediate release of histamine and vasoactive substances but does not involve an immunologic mechanism (non–IgE-mediated). In other words, histamine is released systemically and previous exposure to the offending agent is not required.

In both reactions, the result is respiratory difficulty as a result of bronchoconstriction and possibly pulmonary edema, hypotension through massive vasodilation, edema from increased vascular permeability, shock, and possibly gastrointestinal symptoms. Anaphylactic shock is the most severe type of anaphylaxis and is immediately life-threatening.

Any drug could potentially be associated with an anaphylactic or anaphylactoid reaction. However, the most commonly used chemotherapy drugs associated with anaphylactoid effects are L-asparaginase and doxorubicin. L-asparaginase (a bacterial enzyme) is a foreign protein and can result in an anaphylactic reaction. This is a significant problem in humans (because it is usually given IV) and is uncommon in dogs (usually administered IM or SC). However, an allergic reaction associated with facial edema and pain at the injection site 24 hours later has been reported in dogs. Doxorubicin has infrequently been documented to produce a nonspecific histamine release resulting in a potential increase in serum histamine levels inducing an anaphylactoid reaction manifested as hypotension and tachycardia. There may be an increased risk of this reaction associated with the use of generic doxorubicin.

Other chemotherapy agents have rarely been associated with anaphylactoid reactions. Ifosfamide has been rarely reported to cause this reaction in cats; in dogs and cats, IV etoposide (actually the diluent vehicle polysorbate-80) and IV paclitaxel (actually the diluent vehicle Cremophor-EL) are associated with anaphylactoid reactions severe enough to make some authors suggest these drugs not be used in pet animals.

The route of administration affects the incidence and severity of a reaction. In order of decreasing incidence and severity of associated reactions, they are intravenous, intramuscular, intracavitary, subcutaneous, intradermal, and oral. Other factors known to affect the incidence or severity of hypersensitivity reactions include the class of the drug, the dose, the rate of infusion, the interval between doses, the cumulative dose, the number of previous exposures to the drug, and administration of prophylactic agents (the dosing and timing of administration of the prophylactic agents and the thoroughness of the prevention plan).

## Diagnosis

Anaphylaxis should be assumed and the patient treated accordingly when a patient has a known risk factor (e.g., history of exposure to a drug associated with anaphylaxis), and is showing signs including restlessness, swollen face or legs (Figure 20.1), itchy head, urticaria (Figure 20.2) vomiting/diarrhea, dyspnea, pallor or hypotension.

## Treatment

The three important elements in the treatment of anaphylaxis are early recognition, airway maintenance, and hemodynamic support. Anaphylaxis is generally treated with fluid

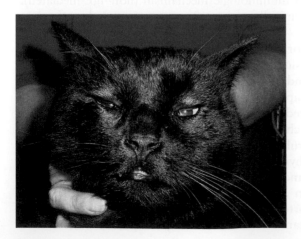

**Figure 20.1.** A cat showing marked facial swelling as an anaphylactoid reaction to ifosfamide chemotherapy. (Courtesy of Dr. Kenneth Rassnick)

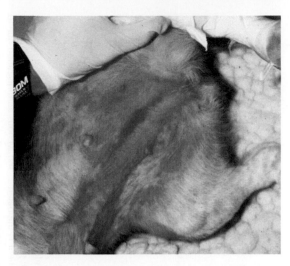

**Figure 20.2.** Severe urticaria on the abdominal skin of a dog receiving etoposide. This is an anaphylactoid reaction to the vehicle diluent, not the chemotherapy itself, and it can be lessened with a slow infusion rate and premedication using corticosteroids and antihistamines. (Courtesy of Dr. Gregory Ogilvie)

therapy (isotonic crystalloid and colloid) to maintain perfusion and blood pressure, as well as a combination of epinephrine, diphenhydramine (antihistamine), and a corticosteroid (dexamethasone, prednisone, methylprednisolone). Epinephrine is recommended because of its inotropic and chronotropic effects on the heart, bronchodilation, and increased intracellular concentrations of cyclic adenosine monophosphate, which decreases synthesis and release of inflammatory mediators of anaphylaxis. However, one study failed to show an improvement in hemodynamics in dogs with anaphylactic shock that were given epinephrine, and it even identified further impairment of left ventricular performance. Recommendations for treatment of anaphylaxis are summarized in Table 20.1.

## Summary: Anaphylaxis

*Causes*

❖ L-Asparaginase
  • **DO NOT USE IV route;** IM or SQ preferred
  • Pretreat with antihistamine ± corticosteroid if patient at risk
❖ Doxorubicin
  • Administered by slow IV under close observation

*Clinical Features*

❖ Client complaint
  • Restlessness
  • Swelling of face or limbs
  • Itchy, red skin (hives)
  • Polydypsia and polyuria
  • Diarrhea

**Table 20.1.** Treatment recommendations for anaphylaxis

| | | | |
|---|---|---|---|
| Discontinue the drug immediately | | | |
| Delay the absorption if possible | | | |
| Oxygen by mask or flow by | | | |
| Patent airway | Intubate if evidence of upper airway obstruction (e.g., laryngeal edema) | | |
| Intravenous isotonic crystalloid (normal saline or lactated Ringer's solution) | 90 ml/kg/hr dogs shock bolus; 50–60 ml/kg/hr cats shock bolus | | |
| Epinephrine | Less severe cases: SQ or IM at a dose of 0.01 mg/kg; repeat at 20 min intervals as needed | More severe cases: 0.01 mg/kg of the 1:10,000 solution given slowly IV (same as 0.1 ml/kg of 1:10,000 IV) | 0.02 mg/kg (0.2 ml/kg of 1:10,000) can be given into the trachea if the patient is intubated and IV access cannot be obtained | Monitor heart rate, rhythm and blood pressure especially with intravenous administration due to potential development of arrhythmias and hypertension (at high dosages) |
| Intravenous colloid (Hetastarch) if hypotension persists | Small incremental boluses of 10 ml/kg/hr in dogs and 6 ml/kg/hr in cats | 1 ml/kg/hr may also be used once the patient has been resuscitated | If a coagulopathy is suspected, blood products, especially fresh frozen plasma, may be necessary: dose of 10–20 ml/kg over several hours (faster if needed for volume resuscitation) |
| Glucocorticoids | 0.5–1 mg/kg IV for dexamethasone sodium phosphate **OR** | 2.0 mg/kg IV prednisolone sodium succinate or methylprednisolone sodium succinate over 20 min | |
| Antihistamine | Diphenhydramine 0.5–1.0 mg/kg SLOW IV (can exacerbate hypotension) or 1.0–2.0 mg/kg IM **OR** | Tripelennamine HCl 1 mg/kg IM (dog, cat) | |

| | | |
|---|---|---|
| H₂ Blocker | cimetidine, ranitidine, and famotidine, can be used to decrease gastric acid secretion stimulated by histamine | Dose varies with each of the H₂ blockers |
| IF HYPOTENSION PERSISTS | Epinephrine CRI 1 ml/kg/hr **OR** 1–10 µg/kg/min: add 4 mg to 1000 ml normal saline (preferred over dopamine in anaphylaxis). Rapid effect, seen within 15 seconds. Decrease rate once BP increases and HR decreases. Slow down if HR increases immediately. Do **NOT** stop infusion suddenly when stable: wean off slowly. | Dopamine 5–10 µg/kg/min CRI; start low, titrate upward |
| IF RESPIRATORY COMPROMISE PERSISTS | Terbutaline 0.01 mg/kg SC or IM | Isoproterenol 0.1–0.2 mg IM dog 0.004–0.006 mg IM cat q 30 min |
| Intense monitoring for 12–24 hr postanaphylaxis | Respiratory rate and rhythm<br>Heart rate and rhythm<br>Blood pressure<br>Pulse oximetry and/or arterial blood gases<br>Urine output<br>PCV and total solids<br>Blood glucose<br>Coagulation parameters<br>Renal values<br>Electrolytes and acid base status<br>Liver values | |

- Vomiting
- Dyspnea, respiratory distress
- Seizures or collapse
- Death

❖ Clinical findings
- Urticaria (hives)and erythema
- Edema (any tissue)
- Pale mucous membranes
- Upper airway obstruction (laryngeal edema)
- Respiratory distress—lower
- Sinus tachycardia
- Dysrhythmia (bradyarrhythmia or tachyarrhythmia)
- Hypotension
- Weak thready pulse
- Vomiting
- Diarrhea (may be hemorrhagic)
- Collapse
- Death

*Diagnostic Findings*

❖ Laboratory
- PCV increased, hemoconcentration (loss of plasma volume due to increased vascular permeability)
- Total solids (TS) reduced (loss of plasma volume)
- Leukocytosis, neutrophilia with left shift
- Eosinopenia initially followed by eosinophilia
- Increased MCV
- Stress hyperglycemia
- Increased clotting times (PT, APTT)
- Increased creatine kinase (CK)
- Increased aspartate aminotransferase (AST)
- Increased alanine aminotransferase (ALT)
- Increased creatinine and blood urea nitrogen (BUN)
- Low pH (acidosis)
- Increased anion gap
- Evidence of DIC (decreased platelets, decreased fibrinogen, increased FDPs, and D-dimer)

❖ ECG
- Sinus tachycardia
- Bradycardia
- Ventricular ectopy or ventricular tachycardia
- Supraventricular tachycardia

❖ Imaging
- Radiography
  ○ Microcardia
  ○ Pulmonary edema—noncardiogenic

*Management*

❖ Depends upon the clinical features upon presentation
❖ Prevention and anticipation (know the drug, the risk, and the patient risk)
  ● Pretreat with antihistamine
  ● Pretreat with corticosteroids
  ● Observe for up to 1 hour posttreatment
❖ Treat systemic anaphylaxis as per Table 20.1.

# Further Reading

Mink SN, et al. 1998. Effect of bolus epinephrine on systemic hemodynamics in canine anaphylactic shock. *Cardiovasc Res* 40:546–556.

Murrant T, Bihari D. 2000. Anaphylaxis and anaphylactoid reactions. *Int J Clin Pract* 54:322–328.

Ogilvie GK, et al. 1994. Prevalence of anaphylaxis associated with the intramuscular administration of L-asparaginase to 81 dogs with cancer: 1989–1991. *J Am Anim Hosp* 4:362–365.

Eschalier A, et al. 1988. Study of histamine release induced by acute administration of antitumor agents in dogs. *Cancer Chemother Pharmacol* 21:246–250.

Phillips BS, et al. 1998. Acute reaction in dogs treated with doxorubicin: Increased frequency with the use of a generic formulation. *J Vet Intern Med* 12:171–172.

# Extravasation Injury

21

*Lee Garrod*

Extravasation is the accidental delivery of any substance outside of the blood vessel into the surrounding subcutaneous or dermal tissue. The agent can escape directly from the vein or the catheter. When the substance is irritant or vesicant, extravasation injury results. The resulting extravasation injury may range from local pain, discomfort, and mild erythema to local tissue damage or moist dermatitis to extensive necrosis.

Several chemotherapy drugs may be classified as vesicants. Commonly used chemotherapy agents that are vesicants include the vinca alkaloids (vincristine, vinblastine, etc.) and the anthracyclines and related drugs (doxorubicin, actinomycin D, etc.). Vincristine and doxorubicin are the most commonly used chemotherapy agents associated with extravasation in veterinary practice.

Vesicants cause an injection site reaction often referred to as a *chemical cellulitis* that initially looks like an irritation but may worsen to irreversible tissue damage leading to severe necrosis. This can start with redness and blistering, but in several days severe skin damage can be evident. Clinical signs may occur 1 to 7 days following extravasation of an irritant; or 7 to 10 days following extravasation of a vesicant such as doxorubicin, and the full extent of injury may not be seen for several weeks. The extent of tissue damage ultimately depends on the concentration, volume, and vesicant nature of the extravasated agent (potency as a reactive chemical that combines with cellular components resulting in cellular changes immediately after exposure).

Cancer patients are inherently at high risk of extravasation because these patients often require multiple venipunctures over time and have thin and fragile veins. In addition, the number of optimal intravenous sites may be reduced due to previous chemotherapy.

Because of the severe consequences of extravasation injury, prevention is critical. Awareness of the specific chemotherapy agents that can be harmful to tissues as well as awareness of risk factors associated with extravasation is key to prevention (see also Chapter 8). Close monitoring of the injection site throughout chemotherapy administration will facilitate immediate recognition of extravasation so that the injection or infusion can be stopped immediately to prevent any further tissue damage.

# Diagnosis

Only a *well-placed clean-stick intravenous catheter* should be used to administer chemotherapy. Do not use IV catheters placed previously for another reason. Administration using a butterfly-winged infusion needle may increase the risk of extravasation. The patient must remain calm and steady throughout the administration of the drug. Extravasation should be suspected if the patient reacts in any way to the drug infusion, the site swells or becomes red, leakage is visualized at the site, resistance occurs when attempting to administer the infusion, or a flash of blood is not obtained on aspiration (however, the presence of blood does not rule out extravasation). If there is any suspicion of extravasation, the treatment must be discontinued immediately. As much of the extravasated substance as possible should be withdrawn through the catheter *before* removing the catheter.

# Treatment

Tissue injury can be extensive if the extravasation goes undetected and untreated. For milder vesicants where the damaged tissue is irritated and necrotic, when the dead tissue sloughs off, it may reveal an ulcer that will eventually heal over about a 6-week period (see Figures 21.1 and 21.2). Doxorubicin is one of the most caustic chemotherapy drugs, and it may continue to destroy tissue relentlessly, despite immediate intervention. The tissue necrosis may spread deeper and expose muscle, tendons, and bone (see Figures 21.3 to 21.7). Even the smallest amount of doxorubicin or actinomycin D can create severe,

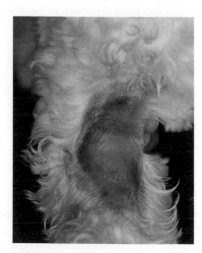

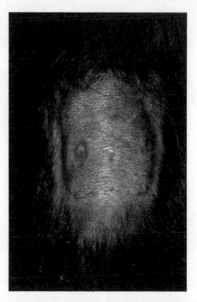

**Figure 21.1.** Vincristine extravasation can lead to pain and swelling if unrecognized at the time of extravasation, or if untreated (as in this dog). Appropriate therapy includes warm compresses, fluid flooding, and hyaluronidase if possible. The patient should be prevented from further injuring the tissue during healing.

**Figure 21.2.** Vincristine extravasation in this dog was unrecognized, but presumably very small, and the majority of damage has come from the patient licking and chewing until small ulcers are created.

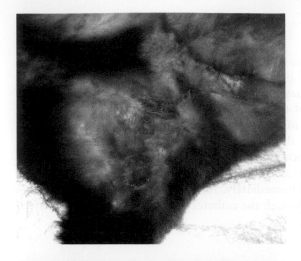

**Figure 21.3.** Doxorubicin extravasation in this cat occurred during a dilute infusion of the drug and was not recognized until the area was flooded. It was treated rapidly with ice compresses, but the slough, while not severe, is extensive and painful.

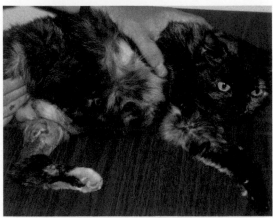

**Figure 21.4.** Doxorubicin extravasation in this cat was less than 0.1 ml of drug, undiluted, and was treated according to recommendations. Despite this treatment, tissue necrosis, swelling, and pain were severe 3 weeks after the incident (see also Figure 21.5). A treatment that could have been considered was surgical excision of the doxorubicin bleb at the time of extravasation.

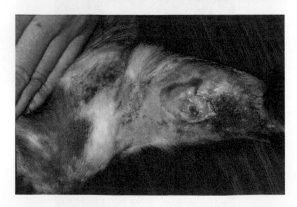

**Figure 21.5.** Closer image of the extravasation injury in Figure 21.4.

irreversible tissue damage. Therefore, extravasation of a drug is treated as a medical emergency and immediate action must be taken.

The rapid treatment of patients with extravasation injury is imperative to improving the outcome. Treatment requires aggressive application of warm (vincristine) or cold (doxorubicin) compresses as often and for as long as the patient will tolerate for at least

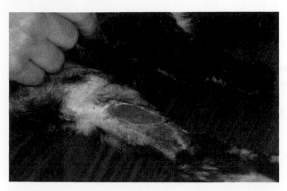

**Figure 21.6.** The same cat as in Figure 21.4, but 6 weeks later, when healing is underway.

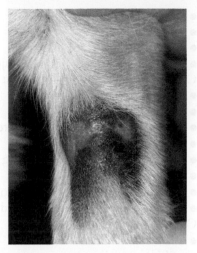

**Figure 21.7.** The healed site of a doxorubicin extravasation showing scarring, contracture, and hyperpigmentation and hypopigmentation. It is no longer painful.

24 hours. In addition, early administration of dexrazoxane for doxorubicin extravasation and hyaluronidase for vincristine extravasation are beneficial. Local application of dimethylsulfoxide (DMSO) is controversial. Despite best efforts, tissue damage may still occur, underscoring the need for prevention.

If tissue damage is extensive, debridement surgery, skin grafting, or even amputation may eventually be required to stop the destruction and resultant pain.

## Summary: Extravasation

*Causes*

- ❖ Vesicant
  - ● Doxorubicin
  - ● Vincristine
  - ● Vinblastine
  - ● Actinomycin D
  - ● *NOTE:* Many other chemotherapy agents may less commonly cause irritation and be vesicants, so care should be taken with all chemotherapy IV infusions.

*Clinical Features*

- ❖ Client complaint posttreatment
  - ● Agitation
  - ● Licking at injection site

- Painful to touch
- Limping
- Redness in area of injection
- Swelling in area or limb of injection
❖ Clinical findings during treatment if suspect extravasation
  - Patient agitated/painful
  - Pruritus
  - Erythema around injection site
  - Swelling
  - Resistance to infusion of drug
  - Reduced flow rate
  - Alarm on infusion pump set off
  - Inadequate flashback of blood
❖ Clinical findings after treatment
  - Moist dermatitis
  - Skin necrosis

## Management

❖ Prevention
  - Blood sampling is done from jugular vein to preserve peripheral veins for injections
  - Do not use existing (previously placed for another reason) catheters for chemotherapy administration
  - Be aware which drugs are extravasation risks, but the best practice is to treat all chemotherapy drugs as risks
  - Proper patient restraint
  - Sedation if restraint is difficult
  - Intravenous catheter rather than butterfly
  - Smallest gauge catheter
  - "Clean-stick" one-time catheter placement
  - Large volume (10 ml) saline flush before and after drug administration
  - Constant observation throughout infusion to completion
    ○ Continuous aspiration of blood throughout administration
❖ If extravasation occurs
  - Discontinue drug administration immediately
  - Notify doctor on duty **IMMEDIATELY**
  - Leave catheter in place
  - Aspirate as much of the drug as possible through the catheter, **AND THEN** remove catheter
    ○ Remove 5 ml blood from cat and 10 ml from dog
  - Doxorubicin
    ○ Ice limb as much as the patient will tolerate for up to 48 to 72 hours
    ○ Dexrazoxane (Zinecard) IV at 10× the mg dose of doxorubicin within 3 hours or 400 to 600 mg/m² IV over 15 minutes; repeat at 24 and 48 hours after extravasation
    ○ Possibly topical dimethylsulfoxide (DMSO) every 8 hours for weeks while assess skin slough

- Vinca alkaloids
  - Infiltrate with 3 to 5 ml 0.9% NaCl
  - Intralesional hyaluronidase total volume equal to extravasated volume of drug in 5 to 6 sites around the edges of lesion with needle changed in between and into patent catheter
  - Warm compress for 15 minutes every 6 hours for 24 hours
- Delayed perivascular damage or slough
  - Daily wound treatment
  - Antibiotics
  - Pain medication
  - Surgical
    - Debridement of tissues
    - Skin grafting
    - Possible amputation

# Further Reading

Bertelli G, et al. 1995. Topical dimethylsulfoxide for the prevention of soft tissue injury after extravasation of vesicant cytotoxic drugs: a prospective clinical study. *J Clin Oncol* 13:2851–2855.

Kisseberth WC, MacEwen EG. 2001. Complications of cancer and its treatment. Adverse effects. In: Withrow SJ, MacEwen EG, eds, *Small Animal Clinical Oncology*, 3rd ed. Philadelphia: W.B. Saunders, 198–218.

Langer SW, et al. 2000. Treatment of anthracycline extravasation with dexrazoxane. *Clin Cancer Res* 6:3680–3686.

Ogilvie GK, Moore AS. 1995. Extravasation of chemotherapy agents. In: Ogilvie GK, Moore AS, eds, *Managing the Veterinary Cancer Patient*. Trenton, Veterinary learning systems, 186–189.

Spugnini EP. 2002. Use of hyaluronidase for the treatment of extravasation of chemotherapeutic agents in six dogs. *J Am Vet Med Assoc* 221:1437–1440.

# Urological Emergencies

*Lee Garrod*

## Acute Renal Failure

Acute renal failure is a medical emergency because it may cause sudden, life-threatening biochemical disturbances. Acute uremia can be classified as one of three categories: prerenal (impaired perfusion of the kidneys), renal (renal tissue damage), and postrenal (obstructive). Renal failure in a cancer patient in particular may be multifactorial. Not surprisingly, prerenal failure is common in this older population. Renal causes related to neoplasia include cancer involving the kidneys or occasionally nephrotoxicity of chemotherapy drugs. Postrenal causes in cancer patients are most commonly neoplasia involving tissue at any level of the urogenital system (obstructive uropathy).

Cancer of the kidney is more common as a cause of acute renal failure in cats than in dogs. When it is present it may be either primary cancer or metastatic cancer originating from another primary tumor. Lymphoma is the most common renal tumor in cats, whereas adenocarcinoma is the most common primary renal tumor in dogs. In cats and dogs with leukemia, the kidneys can be infiltrated with neoplastic cells, which can severely compromise renal function.

Hypercalcemia is a common paraneoplastic syndrome, potentially resulting in calcium nephropathy and renal failure when the calcium × phosphorus product exceeds 70. The hypercalcemia decreases renal blood flow by vasoconstriction. The patient demonstrates polyuria and polydypsia in the early stages of hypercalcemia. Once the calcium x phosphorus product exceeds 70, tissue mineralization ensues, through the binding of calcium and phosphorus, and renal failure can occur.

Patients with neutropenia and sepsis can develop urogenital infection. Infection involving the kidneys, pyelonephritis, results in acute renal failure.

Nephrotoxicity has been associated with some chemotherapy agents in small animals: streptozotocin and cisplatin in dogs (cisplatin is not used in cats due to fatal pulmonary toxicity) and doxorubicin in cats. Cisplatin and streptozotocin are administered using standard, aggressive, saline diuresis protocols, and this dramatically reduces the incidence of nephrotoxicity. Nonsteroidal antiinflammatory medications should be discontinued in patients with existing renal insufficiency.

## Diagnosis

When a patient is presented in renal failure, additional tests may be necessary to exclude other diseases. More than one category of renal failure may be present in an individual patient. Even though cancer or chemotherapy may be in the patient's history, a thorough investigation to rule out the possibility of toxin exposure (ethylene glycol, antifreeze), recent surgery or anesthesia, exposure to nephrotoxic drugs (nonsteroidal antiinflammatory drugs, aminoglycoside antibiotics), or recent illness should be undertaken. Whether acute uremia progresses to acute renal failure depends upon the underlying cause and the early detection and management.

## Treatment

Treatment of acute renal failure starts with careful rehydration and diuresis, monitoring urine output and for evidence of overhydration. Secondary vomiting, electrolyte, acid-base, and biochemical abnormalities should be corrected and controlled as needed. The underlying cause should be corrected whenever possible.

## Summary: Acute Renal Failure

*Causes*

- ❖ Prerenal
    - ● Hypovolemia
        - ○ Dehydration
        - ○ Vomiting
        - ○ Diarrhea
        - ○ Hemorrhage
        - ○ Diuretics
    - ● Hypotension
        - ○ Septic shock
    - ● Decreased renal perfusion
        - ○ Nonsteroidal antiinflammatories (NSAIDS)
        - ○ Angiotensin-converting enzyme inhibitors
- ❖ Renal
    - ● Neoplasia
        - ○ Primary renal neoplasia
        - ○ Metastatic renal neoplasia
        - ○ Paraneoplastic hypercalcemia

- Nephrotoxic chemotherapy
  - Cisplatin (used in dogs only)
  - Methotrexate (high dose or with NSAIDs)
  - Streptozotocin
  - Doxorubicin (cats)
- Glomerulonephritis
- Infection
  - Pyelonephritis
- Renal tubular or tubulointerstitial damage
  - Drugs other than chemotherapy agents
    - Aminoglycosides
    - NSAIDs
    - Radiological contrast agents
  - Ischemia
    - Thrombosis (DIC)
    - Profound hypertension
  - Tumor lysis syndrome
- ❖ Postrenal
  - Obstructive
    - Tumor (transitional cell carcinoma)
    - Calculi
      - Urethral
      - Ureteral
  - Neurologic bladder

*Clinical Features*

- ❖ Client complaint
  - Disorientation
  - Incoordination
  - Lethargy
  - Weakness
  - Depression
  - Decreased urine production
  - Straining to urinate
  - Hematuria
  - Anorexia
  - Polyuria
  - Polydypsia
  - Vomiting
  - Increased respiratory rate
  - Seizures
- ❖ Clinical findings
  - Dehydration
  - Fever
  - Tachycardia
  - Bradycardia (if hyperkalemia)

- Tachypnea
- Hypertension
- Hypotension
- Peripheral edema
- Pulmonary edema

*Diagnostic Findings*

- ❖ Laboratory
  - Complete blood count
    - ○ Anemia
    - ○ Leukocytosis
    - ○ Leukopenia
    - ○ Thrombocytopenia
  - Biochemical profile
    - ○ Uremia
    - ○ Elevated creatinine
    - ○ Hyperphosphatemia
    - ○ Hypercalcemia
  - Electrolytes
    - ○ Hyperkalemia
  - Blood gas analysis
    - ○ Metabolic acidosis
  - Urinalysis
    - ○ Isosthenuria
    - ○ Hematuria
    - ○ Hemoglobinuria or myoglobinuria
    - ○ Pyuria
    - ○ Proteinuria
    - ○ Crystalluria
    - ○ Renal casts
  - Urine culture and sensitivity
  - Urine protein:creatinine ratio
    - ○ Elevated in glomerular disease
  - Coagulation profile
  - Kidney biopsy or fine-needle aspirate
  - Ethylene glycol test
- ❖ ECG
  - Hyperkalemia
    - ○ Bradycardia
    - ○ Loss of P wave
    - ○ Tall peaked T waves
    - ○ Wide QRS complexes
- ❖ Imaging
  - Abdominal radiography
  - Intravenous pyelogram
  - Abdominal ultrasound

- Thoracic radiography
  - ○ Fluid overload/pulmonary edema

*Management*

- ❖ Intravenous crystalloid (0.9% NaCl) fluid
  - Correct dehydration over 6 to 8 hours
    - ○ Watch closely for volume overload
    - ○ Monitor urine output
  - Diuresis after rehydration
    - ○ Can be mild to moderate (2 to 3 × maintenance 66 ml/kg/day) depending on individual patient
- ❖ Monitor urine output
  - Indwelling urinary catheter
    - ○ 2 to 5 ml/kg/hr urine output
  - Measure ins and outs
    - ○ Once a patient is hydrated, ins should match outs
- ❖ Monitor patient for signs of overhydration/volume overload
  - Central venous pressure
  - Heart rate
  - Respiratory rate and lung sounds
  - Weigh patient every 6 hours
- ❖ Control vomiting to reduce ongoing losses
  - Antiemetics
  - Treat gastric hyperacidity with H2-receptor antagonist
  - *NOTE:* Reduce the dose of all drugs that are renally eliminated in patients with reduced renal clearance.
- ❖ Correct electrolyte abnormalities
  - Treatment for hyperkalemia (see Table 19.1)
    - ○ Insulin with 50% dextrose
    - ○ Sodium bicarbonate
    - ○ Calcium gluconate 10% if ECG changes
- ❖ Correct acid-base abnormalities
- ❖ Treatment for hypercalcemia (see Table 19.1)
- ❖ Treatment for hyperphosphatemia
- ❖ Drugs to encourage urine production if oliguric or anuric
  - Mannitol 0.5 to 1.0 gm/kg slow IV
  - Furosemide 2 to 4 mg/kg IV every 1 to 3 hours
  - Dopamine 2 to 3 µg/kg/min CRI
    - ○ Can be used with furosemide
- ❖ Peritoneal dialysis
- ❖ Treatment of neoplasia if underlying cause
- ❖ Management to prevent chemotherapy associated renal damage
  - ○ Saline diuresis according to established protocols for cisplatin and streptozotocin
  - ○ Pretreatment with furosemide (only if well hydrated)
  - ○ Doxorubicin in cats is a cumulative nephrotoxicity; monitor creatinine closely

## Further Reading

Knapp DW, et al. 1988. Cisplatin therapy in 41 dogs with malignant tumors. *J Vet Intern Med* 2:41–46.

Meyer DJ. 1977. Temporary remission of hypoglycemia in a dog with insulinoma after treatment with streptozotocin. *Am J Vet Res* 38:1201–1204.

O'Keefe DA, et al. 1993. Systemic toxicity associated with doxorubicin administration in cats. *J Vet Intern Med* 7:309–317.

## Hematuria

Hematuria is the presence of blood in the urine. Hematuria can be microscopic (detected only on urinalysis) or macroscopic (direct visualization). Seeing blood in the urine of a pet can be alarming to many owners and they perceive it as a true emergency. The hematuria patient in the emergency setting typically presents with the direct visualization of blood in the urine by the owner. There are many potential causes for hematuria, including bacterial infection, bladder wall trauma, urinary crystals or stones, neoplasia of the urogenital system, and coagulopathy.

Often, but not always, the presence of hematuria is associated with straining to urinate (stranguria) (Figure 22.1) and increased frequency of urination (pollakiuria). In a cancer patient, these symptoms certainly could suggest a bacterial cystitis, especially if the patient is immunosuppressed, but it can also be related to recent chemotherapy or other drugs, or even a clotting disorder. Therefore, a complete history alone will often lead to the potential underlying cause. In patients without a prior related history, causes such as cystic calculi, bacterial cystitis, bladder polyps, or urogenital neoplasia, and coagulopathy are all considered.

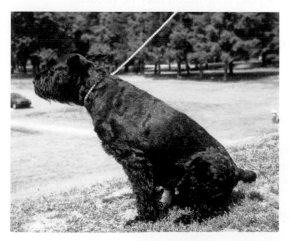

**Figure 22.1.** A dog that is straining to urinate should be investigated with urinalysis, and urine culture and sensitivity, as well as abdominal ultrasonography and possibly cytology or histopathology of any lesions.

Urogenital cancers in dogs most commonly involve the bladder. Transitional cell carcinoma (TCC) is the most common bladder tumor in dogs but is less common in cats. Bleeding due to the presence of a bladder tumor is rarely a life-threatening emergency, because overall blood loss is minimal and the problem is not usually acute in onset. However, some of these patients may have tumor-related obstruction and therefore may have associated renal or electrolyte imbalances that could be life-threatening. Regardless, when presenting as an emergency, diagnostics must be done to evaluate all potential causes.

Hemorrhagic cystitis is a rare complication of certain chemotherapy agents. Cyclophosphamide and ifosfamide can cause sterile hemorrhagic cystitis in the dog. This is due to a direct chemical irritation caused by metabolites to the urothelial (mucosal) lining resulting in inflammation, ulceration, and hemorrhage. The risk of sterile hemorrhagic cystitis is dramatically decreased by the concurrent administration of furosemide during the administration, by diluting irritant metabolites in urine, and by encouraging frequent voiding. In addition, the sulfa drug mesna reduces the risk and severity of sterile hemorrhagic cystitis by binding the irritating metabolites in urine. Dogs receiving cyclophosphamide should have plenty of access to fresh water and opportunity to urinate.

## Diagnosis

The diagnosis of hematuria itself is self-evident. Diagnosis of the underlying cause of hematuria involves urinalysis, urine culture and sensitivity, imaging of the urinary tract, and possibly cytology or histopathology of any lesions. For dogs with a history of cyclophosphamide or ifosfamide administration, urine culture should still be submitted because secondary infections can complicate sterile hemorrhagic cystitis.

## Treatment

Specific treatment is not usually necessary, and treatment depends on the underlying cause. Rarely, if blood loss is severe, transfusion may be needed.

## Summary: Hematuria

*Causes*

- ❖ Urogenital neoplasia
  - ● Malignant
    - ○ Transitional cell carcinoma (97%)
    - ○ Other neoplasia
  - ● Benign
    - ○ Fibroma
    - ○ Leiomyoma
- ❖ Calculi
  - ● Renal
  - ● Ureteral

- Bladder
- Urethral
❖ Chemotherapy agents (sterile hemorrhagic cystitis)
  - Cyclophosphamide
  - Ifosfamide
❖ Glomerulonephritis
❖ Pyelonephritis
❖ Bacterial cystitis
❖ Coagulopathy
❖ Trauma

*Clinical Features*

❖ Client complaint
  - Stranguria
  - Hematuria
  - Pollakiuria
  - Vomiting
  - Anorexia
❖ Clinical findings
  - Hematuria
  - Bladder mass may be palpable (rare) or thick bladder
  - Urethral mass or thickening may be palpable on rectal

*Diagnostic Findings*

❖ Laboratory
  - Urinalysis
    ○ Red blood cells
    ○ White blood cells
    ○ Absence of bacteria
    ○ Proteinuria
    ○ Atypical epithelial cells
  - Urine culture and sensitivity
  - Renal values
  - Coagulation screen
  - Cytology (fine-needle aspirate of a mass) (**Caution:** transitional call carcinoma has been reported to seed along needle tracts)
❖ Imaging
  - Abdominal radiography
  - Abdominal ultrasound
  - Double contrast cystography
  - Thoracic radiographs
    ○ Lung metastases rare with transitional cell carcinoma

*Management*

❖ Antibiotics
❖ Surgery

❖ Treatment for neoplasia
  ● Piroxicam
  ● Chemotherapy
❖ Sterile hemorrhagic cystitis
  ● Prevention
  ● Pain medication
  ● Discontinue chemotherapy drug and change to a different drug
  ● Antibiotics for secondary bladder infection due to bladder wall irritation
  ● Antispasmotic agent oxybutynin 0.2 to 0.3 mg/kg BID to TID
  ● If severe, intravesicular DMSO

## Further Reading

Burnie AG, Weaver AD. 1983. Urinary bladder neoplasia in the dog: A review of seventy cases. *J Small Anim Pract* 24:129–134.

Charney SC, et al. 2003. Risk factors for sterile hemorrhagic cystitis in dogs with lymphoma receiving cyclophosphamide with or without concurrent administration of furosemide: 216 cases (1990–1996). *J Am Vet Med Assoc* 222:1388–1393.

Kisseberth WC, MacEwan EG. 2002. Complications of cancer and its treatment. In: Withrow SJ, MacEwen EG, eds, *Small Anim Clin Oncol*. St. Louis, Elsevier Health Sciences, 198–219.

Phillips BS. 1999. Bladder tumors in dogs and cats. *Comp for Cont Ed Pract Vet* 21:540–547.

# Bone Emergencies

*Lee Garrod*

## Pathologic Fracture

A pathologic fracture is a fracture that occurs through weakened, structurally altered bone. Most pathologic fractures occur in bones affected by cancer. Bones can be affected by either primary or secondary malignancies (metastases). At least 80% of pathologic fractures are due to osteosarcoma.

A pathologic fracture can also occur as a result of other diseases affecting the bone, such as osteomyelitis, bone cyst, or nutritional secondary hyperparathyroidism (osteomalacia).

### Diagnosis

History of sudden onset of non–weight-bearing lameness in a large-breed dog should raise suspicion of pathologic fracture, especially if the dog is known to have a bone tumor. Plain radiographs confirm the presence of a pathologic fracture.

### Treatment

Pathologic fractures cannot easily be repaired. Treatment is directed toward pain management, including amputation where appropriate.

### Summary: Pathologic Fracture

*Causes*

* Primary neoplasia (osteosarcoma)
* Metastatic neoplasia

❖ Osteomyelitis (infection)
❖ Bone cyst
❖ Osteomalacia (nutritional secondary hyperparathyroidism)

*Clinical Features*

❖ Client complaint
  ● Lameness
  ● Pain
❖ Clinical findings
  ● Palpably swollen limb
  ● Palpable fracture

*Diagnostic Findings*

❖ Imaging
  ● Radiography
    ○ Limb radiograph
    ○ Chest radiograph to rule out metastasis

*Management*

❖ Pain management
❖ Amputation
❖ Chemotherapy appropriate for the neoplastic process
❖ Treatment of infectious process if the cause

## Further Reading

Boulay JP, et al. 1997. Pathologic fracture of long bones in the dog. *J Am Anim Hosp Assoc* 23:207–213.

Schneider PR, Stowater JL. 1979. Pathologic fractures associated with skeletal metastasis of osteosarcoma in a dog. *J Am Vet Med Assoc* 175:61–64.

## Hypertrophic Osteopathy

Hypertrophic osteopathy (HO) is a painful debilitating bone disease secondary to disease elsewhere, usually in the thorax. Hypertrophic osteopathy is the most common paraneoplastic disorder associated with primary lung tumors in the dog and cat. Affected animals develop new bone formation on the outside of the diaphyses (shaft) of long bones of the limbs, without destruction of cortical bone.

Hypertrophic osteopathy is usually caused by intrathoracic tumors (primary lung tumors or metastatic; Figures 23.1 and 23.2) or infections (heartworm, Spirocerca, mycobacterium, bacteria, including pulmonary abscess), less commonly by intra-abdominal masses or bladder TCC (Figure 23.3). Affected animals develop bilateral, symmetrical soft tissue

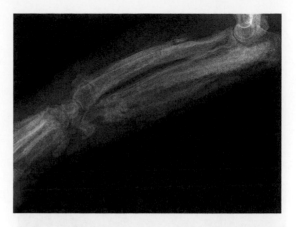

**Figure 23.1.** Hypertrophic osteopathy in a dog with pulmonary metastatic disease. Note the irregular periosteal bone production that affects the radius and ulna, as well as the humerus and metacarpal bones. This condition is often very painful and should prompt thoracic radiographs as a first step to determine a cause.

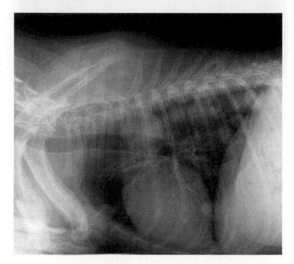

**Figure 23.2.** Pulmonary metastatic disease in the same dog seen in Figure 23.1. Since surgical resection of the multiple masses is impractical, pharmacological palliation of pain would be preferred.

swelling of the lower legs with periosteal new bone formation. These bony changes do not involve the joints or joint capsule. Hypertrophic osteopathy is extremely rare in cats.

## Diagnosis

History of gradual onset of lameness in a dog known to have an intrathoracic tumor suggests HO. Plain radiographs confirm the presence of characteristic periosteal proliferation. If HO is identified before the underlying cause is known, three-view thoracic radiographs are indicated; if this is not productive, abdominal ultrasonography should be done.

## Treatment

Treatment is directed toward pain management and correcting the underlying cause. Surgical removal of the primary tumor usually results in resolution of pain over weeks, followed by slow resolution of radiographic changes.

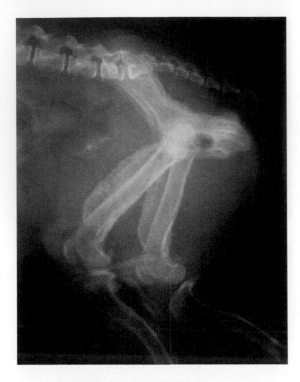

**Figure 23.3.** Rarely, nonpulmonary tumors may be associated with HO; the most commonly reported is urinary bladder transitional cell carcinomas (TCC). In this dog, the bladder TCC is also mineralized, and HO is evident on the pelvis and pelvic limbs. (Courtesy of Dr. Nicole Northrup)

## Summary: Hypertrophic Osteopathy

*Causes*

- ❖ Metastatic pulmonary neoplasia
- ❖ Primary pulmonary neoplasia
- ❖ Pulmonary abscess
- ❖ Bronchopneumonia
- ❖ Bacterial endocarditis
- ❖ Mycobacterium (tuberculosis)
- ❖ Heartworm
- ❖ Spirocercosis
- ❖ Urinary bladder TCC

*Clinical Features*

- ❖ Client complaint
  - ● Asymptomatic
  - ● Stiffness or lameness
  - ● Warm, firm swelling of a limb
  - ● Coughing
  - ● Difficulty breathing
  - ● Exercise intolerance

* Clinical findings
  * Palpably swollen limbs, warm to the touch
  * Pain on palpation of the limbs
  * Abnormal lung sounds

*Diagnostic Findings*

* Imaging
  * Radiography
    * Bilaterally symmetric and generalized periosteal proliferation of long bones
    * Soft tissue swelling with little to no bony abnormality (initial stages)
    * Pulmonary mass or masses

*Management*

* Removal of underlying primary lesion
* Pain medication
* Chemotherapy appropriate for the neoplastic process
* Treatment of infectious process if the cause

# Further Reading

Becker TJ, et al. 1999. Regression of hypertrophic osteopathy in a cat after surgical excision of an adrenocortical carcinoma. *J Am Anim Hosp Assoc* 35:499–505.

Brodey R. 1971. Hypertrophic osteoarthropathy in the dog: A clinicopathologic study of 60 cases. *J Am Vet Med Assoc* 159:1242.

Carrol KB, Doyle L. 1974. A common factor in hypertrophic osteopathy. *Thorax* 29:262–269.

Gerbode F, et al. 1966. Experimental hypertrophic osteopathy. *Surgery* 60:103–112.

Van der Merwe LL, et al. 2008. *Spirocerca lupi* infection in the dog: A review. *Vet J* 176:294–309.

# 24

# Pericardial Effusion and Cardiac Tamponade

*Lee Garrod*

The pericardium is the fibrous membrane that surrounds the heart. Pericardial effusion refers to the presence of fluid in the pericardial space. As the fluid accumulates, it generates pressure on the outside of the heart muscle, and the heart's ability to fill becomes impaired, especially the right atrium and ventricle. There are many causes of pericardial effusion including idiopathic (young dogs), neoplasia, infectious, and rarely traumatic. In cats with congestive heart failure, it is not uncommon to occasionally find a small amount of pericardial effusion, and this is the most common cause of pericardial effusion in this species. The amount in cats is rarely enough to result in clinical symptoms caused by restricted filling.

The most common cause of pericardial effusion in dogs is hemorrhage from a tumor on the right side of the heart, typically the right auricular appendage or right atrium. Of these, hemangiosarcoma is by far the most common neoplasm; and aortic body tumors (chemodectomas) are the second most common neoplasm. Mesothelioma of the pericardial lining itself (primary pericardial neoplasia) can also result in a malignant effusion. Other primary heart tumors can also occur, as well as rare secondary (metastatic) tumors.

Cardiac tamponade occurs when there is excess pericardial effusion, which causes significant compression of the heart itself. The effusion in the majority of cases is blood, but occasionally it can be serosanguinous or purulent. The presence of the fluid in the sac interferes with the filling of the heart, particularly on the right side, and the ventricles collapse. This in turn leads to a decreased stroke volume as well as right-sided congestion (hepatic venous congestion, ascites, pleural effusion). The hemodynamic consequences of the fluid in the pericardial space depend not only on the volume of fluid in the sac but how quickly it has accumulated. If the accumulation has been slow, the pericardium is able to slowly stretch to accommodate the fluid, and a greater volume can be tolerated. A stretched pericardial sac can easily accommodate even 1 liter of fluid.

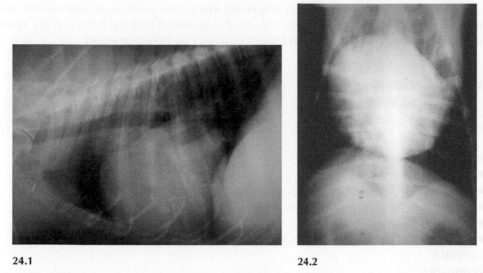

**24.1**                    **24.2**

**Figure 24.1 and Figure 24.2.** Lateral and dorsoventral view of a dog with pericardial effusion. Note the globoid appearance of the heart. Ultrasonography will allow more definitive diagnosis and is the next diagnostic step to consider.

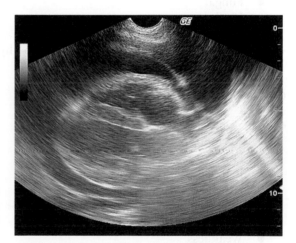

**Figure 24.3.** Ultrasonography demonstrates the pericardial fluid, and can guide collection of a sample for analysis, or therapeutic drainage of the pericardial sac.

## Diagnosis

Pericardial effusion may be suspected based on the history and physical findings. Thoracic radiographs demonstrate cardiomegaly (Figures 24.1 ánd 24.2), and ultrasonography definitively demonstrates fluid in the pericardium (Figure 24.3).

## Treatment

Once the cardiac output becomes severely reduced, the dog ultimately will collapse. Without emergency treatment, the condition is often fatal. Immediate drainage of the pericardial sac is the only treatment to relieve the symptoms associated with cardiac tamponade in an emergency situation. Once the fluid is removed and the heart can fill, restoring adequate cardiac output, other treatment options can be investigated.

## Summary: Pericardial Effusion

*Causes*

* ❖ Malignancy
    * ● Hemangiosarcoma
    * ● Heart base (chemodectoma, ectopic endocrine, hemangiosarcoma)
    * ● Other sarcoma (rhabdomyosarcoma, chondrosarcoma, lymphoma)
    * ● Pericardial (mesothelioma)
    * ● Metastatic (hemangiosarcoma, lymphoma)
* ❖ Idiopathic
* ❖ Traumatic
* ❖ Infection
    * ● Bacterial
    * ● Fungal
    * ● Viral
        * ○ FIP cats
* ❖ Congestive heart failure with cardiomyopathy
    * ● Cats only

*Clinical Features*

* ❖ Client complaint
    * ● Asymptomatic
    * ● Polydypsia
    * ● Inappetence to anorexia
    * ● Difficulty breathing
    * ● Cough
    * ● Exercise intolerance
    * ● Weakness
    * ● Collapse
* ❖ Clinical findings
    * ● Muffled heart sounds
    * ● Pale mucous membranes
    * ● Tachypnea to dyspnea
    * ● Distended jugular veins
    * ● Hypotension
    * ● Tachycardia
    * ● Pulsus paradoxus (weak pulse during inspiration with a stronger pulse during expiration)
    * ● Hepatomegaly
    * ● Signs of right heart failure (ascites, pleural effusion)
    * ● Collapse

*Diagnostic Findings*

❖ Laboratory
  ● No abnormalities
  ● Anemia
  ● Elevated white blood cell count
  ● Uremia
  ● Elevated ALT
  ● Lymphoma
❖ ECG
  ● Diminished QRS voltage
  ● Sinus tachycardia
  ● Electrical alternans
  ● Ventricular ectopy
❖ Imaging
  ● Radiography
    ○ Cardiomegaly
    ○ Enlarged caudal vena cava
    ○ Pleural effusion
    ○ Cardiac mass
    ○ Ascites (decreased abdominal detail)
  ● Echocardiography (image mode preferred)
    ○ Pericardial fluid (small or large volume)
    ○ Cardiac mass
    ○ Heart base mass
    ○ Cardiac tamponade
    ○ Pleural effusion

*Management*

❖ Depends upon the clinical features upon presentation
❖ Sedation and pericardiocentesis when:
  ● Cardiac tamponade
  ● Respiratory distress
  ● Pleural effusion
  ● Significant abdominal effusion
  ● Weakness or collapse
  ● Diagnostic sample required for analysis
❖ Thoracentesis if symptomatic for pleural effusion (rare)
❖ Supportive treatment with IV fluids to help the heart fill (judicious if left-sided failure has also developed)
❖ Diuretic low dose if excessive ascites or pleural effusion
❖ ECG monitoring
❖ Surgery
  ● Cardiac tumor/auricular appendage resection
  ● Pericardial window
  ● Subtotal pericardectomy
  ● Percutaneous balloon pericardiotomy

# Further Reading

Guglielmini C, et al. 2007. Metastatic pericardial tumors in a dog with equivocal pericardial cytological findings. *J Am Anim Hosp Assoc* 43:284–287.

Hall DJ, et al. 2007. Pericardial effusion in cats: a retrospective study of clinical findings and outcomes in 146 cats. *J Vet Intern Med* 21:1002–1007.

Ogilvie GK, Moore AS. 1995. *Managing the Veterinary Cancer Patient*, 1st ed. Trenton, Veterinary Learning Systems Co., Inc, 441–444.

Ware WA, Hopper DL. 1999. Cardiac tumors in dogs: 1982–1995. *J Vet Intern Med* 13:95–103.

# Section 7

## Common Cancers in Veterinary Patients

# Lymphoma in Dogs

25

## Overview

Lymphoma, or lymphosarcoma, is a cancer seen in many species of animals and in humans. Lymphoma is the malignant proliferation of lymphocytes, which are a major component of the immune system. Most often, a pet's caregiver will notice enlarged lymph nodes. Less commonly the dog may have a reduced appetite and less energy. Diagnosis is normally based on a lymph node biopsy, thoracic and abdominal radiographs, and standard blood tests and urinalysis, but may also include more complicated procedures such as bone marrow evaluation.

Lymphoma is caused by a variety of factors, potentially involving genetic components, exposure to carcinogens, and other unknown factors. Although the **lymph nodes** are often the most obvious to a caregiver, **other organs** of the body, including liver, spleen, and bone marrow, may become affected, and the function of normal cells may be compromised. For example, liver damage may occur because of the expanding tumor cell population in the liver causing elevations in serum ALT and ALP, and in severe cases, patients may have liver dysfunction. Normally the bone marrow produces the majority of the blood cells. Tumor cells in the bone marrow can cause fewer neutrophils or platelets to be available. The pet is then susceptible to infection and bleeding (petechiation or ecchymoses). Anemia is commonly low-grade and due to "chronic disease" rather than bone marrow infiltration.

The affected pet may develop **paraneoplastic syndromes** or tumor-associated conditions. For example, there may be abnormal proteins (hyperglobulinemia) or hypercalcemia due to secondary effects of the lymphoma. These syndromes themselves can cause acute, life-threatening problems; and careful monitoring is important.

For lymphoma in dogs, remission times and life span, or **prognosis**, is highly variable and depends on a number of factors:

1. *Immunophenotype:* whether the lymphocyte cell type is T- or B-cell. Dogs with B-cell type do better than those with T-cell type. This must be tested on biopsy by immunohistochemistry.
2. *Substage:* whether the pet is feeling ill. Loss of appetite is probably the most important symptom in this regard (Figures 25.1 and 25.2). Dogs in substage a (no symptoms) do better than dogs in substage b (feeling unwell or having high blood calcium).
3. The *stage* of the disease, which reflects the number and location of major populations of tumor cells in the body. Stage 3 means all lymph nodes affected. Stage 5 is the highest. Dogs with stage 1 and 2 do better than dogs with higher stages (Figures 25.3 and 25.4).
4. *Histologic grading:* the specific appearance of tumor cells and their pattern of infiltration in various tissues (what the pathologists reports from a biopsy specimen).

### Dogs in Substage a Live Longer than Dogs in Substage b

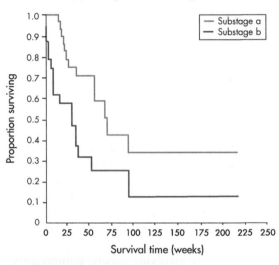

**Figure 25.1.** Kaplan-Meier survival curve showing dogs in substage a (physically well) live longer than dogs in substage b (clinical signs of illness). Keller et al., *J Vet Internal Med* 7:289–295, 1993, with permission (from *Managing the Canine Cancer Patient,* Veterinary Learning Systems 2006, with permission).

### Anorexia Predicts Shorter Remission Duration

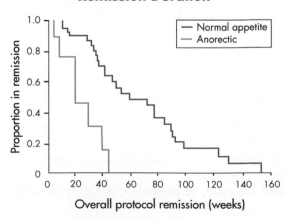

**Figure 25.2.** Kaplan-Meier survival curve showing that dogs eating normally live longer than dogs that are anorectic. Moore et al., *J Vet Internal Med* 15:348–354, 2001, with permission (from *Managing the Canine Cancer Patient,* Veterinary Learning Systems 2006, with permission).

Clinical stages of canine lymphoma

| Clinical Stage* | Criteria |
| --- | --- |
| Stage 1 | Involvement limited to single node or lymphoid tissue in single organ (excluding the bone marrow) |
| Stage 2 | Regional involvement of many lymph nodes, with or without involvement of the tonsils |
| Stage 3 | Generalized lymph node involvement |
| Stage 4 | Involvement of liver and/or spleen, with or without generalized lymph node involvement |
| Stage 5 | Involvement of blood, bone marrow, and/or other organs |

*Stages are further classified to clinical substage a (no clinical signs) or b(with clinical signs). For example, Stage IIIa describes a dog with generalized lymphadenopathy and no clinical signs.

**25.3**

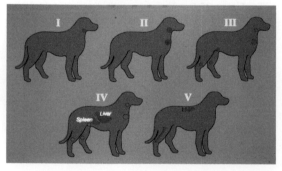

**25.4**

**Figure 25.3 and Figure 25.4.** A tabular (25.3) and a visual schematic (25.4) (from *Managing the Canine Cancer Patient,* Veterinary Learning Systems 2006, with permission) describing the stages of lymphoma in dogs.

5. The *presence of paraneoplastic syndromes* (see above).
6. The *treatment* chosen and the *care* given by the owner and veterinary cancer care team.
7. The *individual pet's response* to therapy.

## Diagnosis and Staging

Lymphoma is suspected based on physical examination (Figures 25.5 and 25.6) and is best confirmed on histopathology; cytology is usually suggestive but not definitively diagnostic.

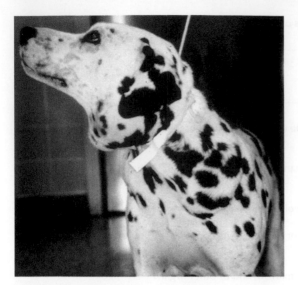

**Figure 25.5.** A 6-year-old female Dalmatian with massive peripheral lymphadenopathy, but no clinical illness and no other sites of lymphoma on staging. The lymphoma is therefore classified as stage 3a. Immunophenotyping will help define the best recommendation for treatment.

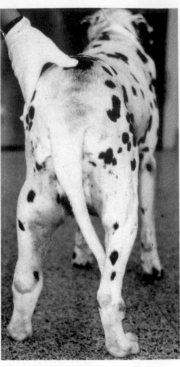

**Figure 25.6.** The same patient as in Figure 25.5; note the hindlimb edema caused by the massive lymph node enlargement.

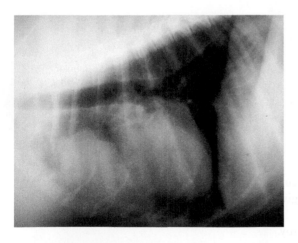

**Figure 25.7.** A lateral thoracic radiograph shows an anterior mediastinal lymphoma. These are often seen as part of T-cell lymphoma in dogs and commonly associated with hypercalcemia. (Courtesy of Kenneth M. Rassnick)

Immunophenotyping should be requested on a biopsy (the tests to ask for are B-cell (CD-79) and T-cell (CD-3) stains.

Dogs with lymphoma should be staged using thoracic radiographs (Figure 25.7) (lymphadenopathy, pleural effusion or pulmonary infiltration all affect quality of life and clinical management). Abdominal radiographs or ultrasonography can be used to evaluate the liver and spleen in dogs where the abdomen is difficult to palpate. CBC, serum chemistry profile, and urinalysis should be performed, and bone marrow aspiration cytology should be considered for dogs that have cytopenias on their CBC (other than anemia of chronic disease).

In general, dogs with a lower stage of lymphoma, dogs that are not sick (substage a) and dogs that have a B-lymphocyte derived tumor have a better chance of remission with treatment.

## Treatment

Untreated dogs usually live 2 months or less. The treatment of lymphoma has evolved to parallel the treatment of the disease in humans, with certain differences. The goal of chemotherapy is to achieve a complete **clinical remission** (CR), which means to make the pet feel as normal as possible with no outward evidence of cancer. The enlarged lymph nodes decrease in size and symptoms disappear for the duration of the remission. With therapy, most dogs with lymphoma live 9 months to 1 year or more. Therefore, a reasonable goal is a 1-year survival. Occasionally a dog will live much longer, up to 2.5 years or more, and about 15% of dogs with lymphoma are permanently cured by combination chemotherapy.

Treatment usually involves the use of multiple anticancer chemotherapy drugs, some used simultaneously and others in sequence. They are used in a set format, or **protocol**. Various such protocols exist, using slightly different drug sequences and dosages. In general, similar remission time and life span are achieved with all protocols that use the same drugs, so that one is not necessarily "better" than another. However, it is important to use different drugs in combination, since this has been shown to dramatically increase remission time. The most effective, and commonly used, drugs are vincristine, cyclophosphamide, prednisone, L-asparaginase, and doxorubicin.

There are several specific **phases of chemotherapy** in the treatment of lymphoma. Treatment always begins with the **induction** phase, and the other phases are used in particular situations. During induction, aggressive chemotherapy is initiated in order to kill as many tumor cells as rapidly as possible without causing severe side effects. The goal of the induction phase is to induce a complete remission. This is most likely to occur with an induction phase involving the five drugs listed above. A complete blood count (with particular attention to the absolute neutrophil count) is measured weekly during this phase to make sure there are enough cells to fight off infections as well as platelets for clotting. The **consolidation** phase is used in some protocols to bring induction to a close. Toward the end of induction, the number of tumor cells is hopefully very low. Consolidation is designed to theoretically eliminate the remaining lymphoma cells. This is often not entirely possible; there are nearly always a few left even after this aggressive step is taken because of the lower dosages used in veterinary chemotherapy than those used when treating human patients.

The **maintenance** phase of chemotherapy usually follows consolidation. The goal is to keep the pet in complete remission while decreasing the potential risk of side effects from continuous use of potent, high-dose anticancer drugs. This should decrease the amount of drugs required to keep the pet in remission by reducing the frequency of administration. It is important for caregivers to observe their pet closely for any adverse signs that could signal relapse. These signs are usually similar to the original signs the dog had before receiving therapy, but occasionally new signs can arise. Recent changes to chemotherapy protocols are attempting to reduce the maintenance phase of treatment in order to improve the pet's quality of life and the amount of chemotherapy it will receive. Intermittent use of "induction" treatments appears to be as good as using continual "maintenance" chemotherapy for some pets and their caregivers.

**Rescue** is a term used for aggressive therapy needed when the lymphoma no longer responds to the routine chemotherapy protocol. Over time, the tumor cells may become resistant to the drugs being used and again multiply to a critical number, causing signs such as reenlargement of lymph nodes, lethargy, etc. At this point, new drugs or higher dosages are needed to reinduce a remission. Many times this is successful and the pet may again do well for some time. However, with each successive relapse it becomes more difficult to reinduce remission until finally the disease become resistant to treatment. Drugs used in this setting include lomustine, mechlorethamine (mustargen) and procarbazine. These drugs are alkylating agents and usually have no cross-resistance with drugs used in first-line therapy for lymphoma in dogs.

## Nursing Highlights

One of the very important roles for veterinary technicians/nurses in this disease is emphasizing to owners that delaying starting treatment until their pet "needs it" is not a good strategy. In various studies dogs with lymphoma that are unwell (substage b) at the start of therapy have median remission times approximately half of those reported for "well" dogs (substage a). More specific symptoms may predict outcomes even more accurately. In one study, of dogs eating normally before diagnosis, 90% achieved complete remission; of dogs with inappetence, only 60% achieved complete remission. Even when a patient's history indicates it has been well, it is important to start therapy before such symptoms arise. It is important to stress to owners that delaying starting treatment until their pet is are sick will make it more difficult to treat successfully. Supportive care can improve both the remission rate and survival time for unwell dogs.

Technicians/nurses are often asked by owners for guidance in deciding about the benefits or otherwise of chemotherapy. It is important to recognize that although they are dealing with a rarely curable disease, their pet can be treated in such a way that a **high quality of life** is achieved. In this respect, it is similar to treating heart or kidney disease, which can also be fatal eventually but which can be managed for some time with a good quality of life.

Many pet owners wonder whether they should feed their pet anything special during treatment for lymphoma. There is some evidence that higher protein and fat and lower carbohydrate content is beneficial to dogs with lymphoma. A commercially available canned food for dogs that follows these principles and is supplemented with additional nutrients that may benefit dogs with lymphoma is Hill's Prescription diet n/d, but homemade diets such as that in Figure 12.3, may also provide a similar benefit. Again, quality of life is the most important criterion for pets undergoing treatment for cancer, and it is important that the diet chosen is one that the patient enjoys.

## Case Example

Hannah, an 8-year-old, spayed female, 26.8 kg German shepherd was noted by her owner to have "masses under her neck" and examination by her veterinarian confirmed markedly enlarged peripheral lymph nodes (submandibular, prescapular, inguinal, and popliteal) with no associated clinical signs of illness. This presentation is classical for lymphoma, and biopsy of a lymph node was appropriately performed. The diagnosis was high-grade diffuse lymphoblastic lymphoma. Immunophenotype was B-cell. CBC and chemistry panel were normal. Thoracic radiographs showed only mild pulmonary consolidation (felt to be age rather than disease-related). Based on these results, she was considered to be in at least clinical stage 3, substage a.

### Further Staging

Baseline lymph node measurements should be recorded to evaluate response to treatment.

In addition to the already performed CBC and chemistry panel, urinalysis (with culture, if indicated) is recommended to detect any subclinical UTI, common in dogs with lymphoma.

Careful abdominal palpation, and radiography or ultrasonography if the liver and spleen cannot be clearly palpated as normal, is indicated. Hepatic or splenic involvement elevates the stage to 4.

A careful physical examination of her cardiovascular system should be done, and if there is any question of abnormality, baseline cardiac ultrasonography is indicated. If ultrasonography shows any evidence at all of ventricular dilation or reduced shortening fraction, doxorubicin is contraindicated.

### Case Resolution

Hannah was a very typical lymphoma patient and she was felt to be likely to have a very good response to chemotherapy. Further staging revealed no abnormalities and chemotherapy was started with a five-drug protocol using the drugs listed above. She achieved a complete remission by her third week of treatment and finished her protocol. Relapse was noted at a regular examination 9 months later, and repeated treatment caused a second remission. At her second relapse 5 months later, rescue therapy using lomustine, actinomycin-D, and procarbazine was prescribed because the other drugs she had been receiving were no longer effective, and a third remission was achieved for another 3 months. Her total survival time was 2 months longer than that, and her owner was very pleased with the additional 2 years of good quality of life.

# Lymphoma in Cats

26

## Overview

Lymphoma, or lymphosarcoma, is a cancer seen in many species of animals and in humans. Lymphoma is the malignant proliferation of lymphocytes, which are a major component of the immune system. Cats with lymphoma are usually unwell, with extranodal (other than lymph node) sites more commonly affected than lymph nodes. The most commonly involved system is the gastrointestinal tract (Figure 26.1). Often cats are presented for reduced appetite and less energy and diagnosis is made during investigation. Diagnosis is normally based on a biopsy, thoracic radiographs (Figure 26.2) and abdominal ultrasonography (often used to direct the biopsy), and standard blood tests and urinalysis, but may also include more complicated procedures such as CT scan or cytology of other sites (Figure 26.3).

Lymphoma in cats is caused by a variety of factors. The best studied is feline leukemia virus (FeLV); more recently FeLV has been found to be an uncommon cause of lymphoma, probably due to testing and isolation of infected cats leading to a decreased prevalence. In the 2000s other causes predominate, including genetic components (Oriental breeds are at higher risk), exposure to carcinogens (cats exposed to second-hand smoke are 3 to 4 times more likely to develop lymphoma), and other unknown factors. Because multiple organs may become affected, including kidney, gastrointestinal tract, and central nervous system, as well as the liver and bone marrow, the function of normal cells may be compromised. For example, renal damage may occur because of the expanding tumor cell population in the kidney causing elevations in serum creatinine and urea, and in severe cases, patients may have renal failure. Normally the bone marrow produces the majority of the blood cells. Tumor cells in the bone marrow can cause fewer neutrophils or platelets to be available. The pet is then susceptible to infection and bleeding (petechiation or ecchymoses). Anemia is commonly low-grade and due to "chronic disease" rather than bone marrow infiltration.

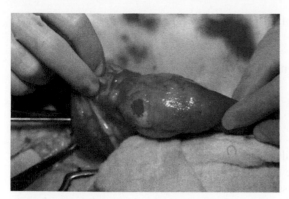

**Figure 26.1.** A 13-year-old spayed female DLH with a history of anorexia and vomiting. Physical examination showed cachexia, and abdominal palpation was suggestive of an intra-abdominal mass. Exploratory laparotomy confirmed the presence of this intestinal mass, and histopathology showed it to be lymphoma. (Courtesy of John Berg)

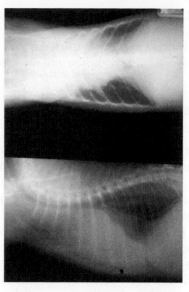

**Figure 26.2.** A 10-year-old neutered male Burmese with a history of weight loss and dyspnea. Thoracic radiographs showed a large cranial mediastinal mass. (Courtesy of Susan M. Cotter)

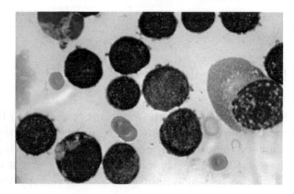

**Figure 26.3.** Cytology of the cranial mediastinal mass seen in the patient in Figure 26.2; the presence of a highly variable population of large lymphoblasts is strongly suggestive of lymphoma. (Courtesy of Susan M. Cotter)

For lymphoma in cats, remission times and life span, or **prognosis**, is highly variable and depends on a number of factors:

1. The *stage* of the disease, which reflects the number and location of major populations of tumor cells in the body. Stage 5 is the highest. Cats with stage 1 lymphoma do better than cats with higher stages.
2. *Substage:* whether the pet is feeling ill. Loss of appetite is probably the most important symptom in this regard since cats can lose a large percentage of their body weight in a very short time. Cats in substage a (no symptoms) do better than cats in substage b (feeling unwell). Unfortunately, most cats are substage b when diagnosed.
3. *Histologic grading:* the specific appearance of tumor cells and their pattern of infiltration in various tissues (what the pathologist reports from a biopsy specimen).

Low-grade lymphoma is better, and often requires less aggressive therapy to gain a similar remission.
4.  The *pet's response* to therapy.
5.  The *treatment* chosen and the *care* given by the owner and veterinary cancer care team.

## Treatment

Treatment usually involves the use of multiple anticancer chemotherapy drugs in a set format, or **protocol**. It is important to use different drugs in combination, since this has been shown to dramatically increase remission time. The most effective, and commonly used, drugs are vincristine, cyclophosphamide, prednisone, procarbazine, and doxorubicin. L-asparaginase is much less effective in cats than in dogs.

In general, cats with a lower stage of lymphoma and cats that are not sick have a better chance of remission with treatment. Untreated cats usually live 2 months or less. With therapy, approximately 50% of cats with lymphoma achieve a remission (lower than for dogs), and live 1 year or more (the same as dogs). Therefore, a reasonable goal is a 1-year survival. Occasionally a cat will live much longer, up to 2.5 years or more, and about 20% of cats with lymphoma are permanently cured by combination chemotherapy.

More commonly in cats than in dogs, a truly localized (stage 1) lymphoma may be found. Often this involves the nasal cavity, but it can involve other sites. For these patients, localized therapy (surgery or radiation therapy) may provide a valuable adjunct to chemotherapy; or even be used alone (as long as there is not evidence of systemic lymphoma on staging). The prognosis for stage 1 lymphomas is favorable.

## Nursing Highlights

Supportive care is often important for cats with lymphoma involving the gastrointestinal tract. Any progression of GI signs means that the patient will need nutritional support. Some of the chemotherapeutics have the potential to make these symptoms worse. Cats may lose a large percentage of their body weight in even as short a period as a week, and continued loss of weight after staring therapy should be considered unacceptable. Antiemetics (metoclopramide) and appetite stimulants (such as megestrol acetate or cyproheptadine orally) may be appropriate in addition to good general nursing care in order to improve nutritional status if chemotherapy is used. Placement of an esophagostomy, gastrostomy, or pharyngeal feeding tube is essential in cats with marked GI signs. In addition to assisting in feeding, this tube will also enhance the caregiver's ability to administer oral medication. The use of prophylactic antibiotics should be considered, particularly when administering a myelosuppressive drug for the first time.

Many pet owners wonder whether they should feed their pet anything special during treatment for lymphoma. There is some evidence that higher protein and fat and lower carbohydrate content is beneficial to dogs with lymphoma, but similar studies have not been performed in cats. Cats have special nutritional requirements, and Hill's Prescription diet n/d is not a suitable diet for cats. Since quality of life is the most important criterion for pets undergoing treatment for cancer, it is important that the diet chosen is one that the patient enjoys.

# Case Example

Blue, an 11-year-old castrated male, 5 kg DSH had a history of sneezing beginning approximately 3 months before presentation and gingivitis for which he received dental care with extractions. Following that intervention he had become inappetent and required supportive care. He was serologically negative for FeLV and FIV. His CBC was unremarkable, and the only abnormality on the serum biochemistry panel was an elevated globulin level. Nasal radiographs demonstrated a soft tissue mass in the left nasal sinus. Nasopharyngoscopy demonstrated a smooth fleshy mass that was biopsied for histopathology and yielded a diagnosis of high-grade lymphoma (frequent mitoses and extensive regions of coagulative necrosis).

Blue was thought to have a stage 1 (localized) lymphoma. Further testing was performed to confirm this because cats that have multiorgan involvement found on further testing have a worse prognosis and require more aggressive treatment. The best treatment is usually *combination chemotherapy and radiation therapy*. Chemotherapy alone is not as effective as radiation for the treatment of local disease (radiation killing is not limited by systemic toxicity), but radiation alone should be used only if *exhaustive* staging has failed to demonstrate any other site of lymphoma (hence the somewhat aggressive staging recommendations).

## Further Staging

The abdomen and thorax should be evaluated by abdominal ultrasonography and thoracic radiographs, respectively (with aspiration cytology or biopsy of any lesions seen).

For completeness, if radiation therapy alone is being considered, bone marrow cytology should be evaluated for lymphoma.

Urinalysis should be evaluated for subclinical infection, but also for concentrating ability, which may determine the safety of doxorubicin chemotherapy. Of particular concern would be if his specific gravity is <1.030. Serum T4 should be evaluated because hyperthyroidism may mask renal insufficiency.

Immunophenotype may have prognostic value for cats with lymphoma, so stains for B- (CD-79a) and T-cell (CD-3) markers on the biopsy should be considered.

If radiation therapy is being considered, a CT scan is needed to delineate the treatment field. This will also allow examination of the cribriform plate, an important prognostic factor in a recent study.

## Case Resolution

Blue's staging showed that he had normal renal function, and there was no evidence of lymphoma on further staging. Radiotherapy was not an option for this owner, and Blue began receiving chemotherapy on a combination chemotherapy protocol. He initially experienced a strong (80%) partial response to chemotherapy, but symptoms returned in the third week of therapy. Nasal bacterial culture was positive, and the signs again subsided with appropriate antibiotic therapy. Chemotherapy was continued and 6 months after treatment began, a repeated CT scan showed no evidence of lymphoma. All treatment was ceased and 2 years later he was still free of signs of disease.

# 27

# Mast Cell Tumor in Dogs

## Overview

Mast cells are normally found throughout the body and are considered part of the allergy system because they contain histamine and other substances that cause swelling and itchiness when released from the cell. **Mast cell tumors (MCT)** are one of the most common skin tumors in dogs and range from essentially benign to highly malignant. The most reliable predictor of how an individual mast cell tumor will behave is the **grade** of the tumor, which is determined by biopsy:

1. **Grade 1** MCT are benign, usually quite small, and localized to the superficial skin layers. They are usually **cured** by wide surgical removal that includes a "cuff" of normal tissue both around and below the tumor.
2. **Grade 2** MCT are **locally invasive** (meaning they invade adjacent normal tissue), but they do not typically spread to other places in the body, particularly if they are treated appropriately early in the course of the tumor. In this respect they are "between" grade 1 and grade 3 tumors.
3. **Grade 3** MCT are often very large, often (but not always) associated with swelling and pain and may spread rapidly to other sites in the body. These tumors are **difficult** to control (Figure 27.1).

A recent study also found that the mitotic index (number of mitoses counted per 10 high-power microscope fields [HPF]) predicted survival for dogs that had grade 2 or 3 MCT. Dogs with MCT with a mitotic index of <5 had long survival times of more than 5 years, compared to 2–4 months if the mitotic index was >5.

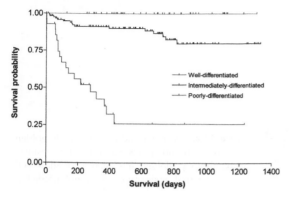

**Figure 27.1.** Kaplan-Meier survival curve showing the effect of tumor grade on survival for dogs with mast cell tumors. Murphy et al., *Vet Rec* 158:287–291, 2006, with permission.

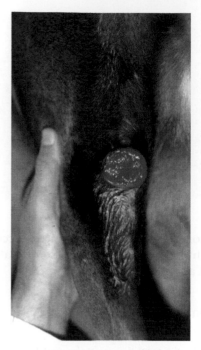

**Figure 27.2.** A 9-year-old spayed female Weimaraner with an ulcerated mass on the caudal aspect of the left stifle; histopathology yielded a diagnosis of mast cell tumor. (Courtesy of A. G. Evans)

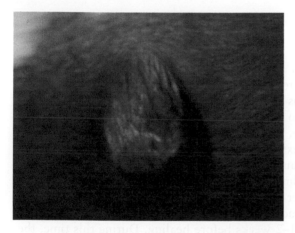

**Figure 27.3.** Another mass on the same patient as in Figure 27.1; histopathology also yielded a diagnosis of mast cell tumor. The presence of multiple tumors does not in itself confer a worse prognosis, and each tumor should be treated individually. (Courtesy of A. G. Evans)

## Diagnosis and Staging

The diagnosis of MCT may be suspected by physical examination, but any cutaneous lesion could be an MCT, and diagnosis cannot be predicted by external appearance (Figures 27.2–27.4). Diagnosis of MCT can often be made by FNA cytology; however, histopathology is necessary for the critically important information of tumor grade.

Staging for dogs with MCT is performed to check for MCT spread to the most commonly affected sites: lymph nodes (the most common site), bone marrow, or abdominal organs such as spleen and liver. Radiographs, abdominal ultrasonography, and bone marrow aspirate may need to be performed in addition to CBC, serum biochemistry profile, and urinalysis. Buffy coat smears are no longer considered helpful in staging dogs with MCT.

Even after successful treatment of an MCT, about 10% of dogs will develop **another** skin MCT, months to years later. Most oncologists believe this is unrelated to the original

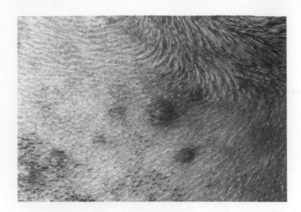

**Figure 27.4.** A 6-year-old castrated male golden retriever with multiple small cutaneous lesions; histopathology yielded a diagnosis of mast cell tumor. External appearance does not predict a diagnosis.

tumor, and can often be treated successfully. Early detection will help in the successful treatment of second tumors, so the patient should be carefully evaluated at each examination and by their owner.

## Treatment

Grade 1 MCT is usually cured by surgery.

Treatment of grade 2 MCT with low mitotic index is primarily aimed at controlling the tumor where it occurs because metastasis is uncommon. There are generally two means of achieving this control. The first is **surgery** to remove the MCT and a wide and deep (usually 2 cm) margin of normal surrounding tissue, which can be difficult depending on where the tumor is on the body. Particularly on the extremities (leg, face, etc.) it may not be possible to completely remove all the tumor cells, and the MCT will regrow. The second option is **radiation therapy**. Radiation therapy is administered to the tumor and a similar 2 cm cuff of normal tissue, but normal tissue is better able to repair the damage caused by radiation therapy than is the tumor. Side effects of radiation therapy include a skin burn that develops midway through treatment and lasts 1–2 weeks before healing. During this time, the pet should be treated with oral antiinflammatory and analgesic medications and topical burn creams to minimize discomfort. There is also the potential, though very unlikely, for permanent damage to underlying tissues depending on the location of the tumor. With radiation therapy, there is a 95% chance of controlling the tumor for 1 year and an 80–95% chance of controlling the tumor long-term (cure); this is very similar to surgery.

If the MCT is grade 3 or grade 2 with a high mitotic index, **chemotherapy** should be considered.

## Nursing Highlights

Dogs with larger, bulky MCT disease, with recurrence of cutaneous disease, or with systemic spread of MCT, should receive $H_2$ antagonists, because rapid degranulation of neoplastic mast cells may follow surgery or chemotherapy. The objective is to prevent gastrointestinal ulceration associated with elevated levels of histamine and to treat ulcers already present. $H_2$ antagonists such as ranitidine or famotidine reduce gastric acid production by competitive inhibition of the action of histamine on $H_2$ receptors of the gastric parietal cells. Omeprazole, which inhibits gastric acid production by the gastric parietal cells through proton pump inhibition, may also be used. Dogs with evidence of gastrointestinal ulceration and bleeding may benefit from sucralfate therapy. Sucralfate reacts with stomach acid to form a highly condensed, viscous, adherent, pastelike substance that binds to the surface of both gastric and duodenal ulcers. The barrier formed protects the ulcer from potential ulcerogenic properties of pepsin, acid, and bile, allowing the ulcer to heal. $H_1$ antagonists (e.g., diphenhydramine) should be considered for use along with an $H_2$ antagonist before and after surgical removal of canine MCTs to help prevent the negative effects of local histamine release on fibroplasia and wound healing.

## Case Example

Emma, a 7-year-old, spayed female, 30 kg bull terrier had a grade 2 MCT excised with complete histologic margins from the proximal cranial portion of the left hindleg. Prior to surgery, a CBC and serum chemistry profile showed no significant abnormalities that would interfere with further treatment. The regional popliteal inguinal and sublumbar lymph nodes were not enlarged, and no other cutaneous masses were reported. The mitotic index of the excised MCT was reported as 10 per 10 HPF, which was suggestive of aggressive biologic behavior.

### Further Staging

Ultrasonography is recommended to evaluate the sublumbar (iliac) lymph nodes.

The abdomen should be carefully palpated, and if there is difficulty palpating the organs clearly or if there is any suspicion of hepato- or splenomegaly, these organs should be evaluated further by ultrasound-guided fine-needle aspiration cytology.

Thoracic radiographs are usually considered part of routine staging of pets with cancer. Pulmonary involvement with MCT is uncommon, so these may be "low yield" in staging this disease; but other abnormalities such as sternal lymphadenopathy, or other intercurrent disease, could be identified.

Approximately 5% of dogs have mast cell infiltration of the bone marrow. Because of the high-grade histology, and if aggressive chemotherapy is being considered, this would be a worthwhile test, because it may change the perception of tumor burden before chemotherapy but would not change the treatment used.

### Case Resolution

Further staging showed Emma had metastasis to the sublumbar lymph nodes, and since surgery had resulted in complete margins, radiation therapy was not felt to offer any advantage for local tumor control. It was felt that the treatment most likely to result in long tumor control would be adjuvant chemotherapy, and a protocol including CCNU, vinblastine, and prednisone was prescribed. Complete response was seen in the lymph nodes, but Emma developed persistent liver enzyme elevation after her second dose of CCNU, and this drug was discontinued because it is a potential hepatotoxin. However, vinblastine and prednisone were continued. She was still free of evidence of cancer 8 months later.

# Soft Tissue Sarcomas in Dogs and Cats

## Overview

Soft tissue sarcomas (STS) are a group of tumors that arise from connective tissues such as fibrous tissue and muscle. Some of the specific tumors in this category are fibrosarcomas, neurofibrosarcomas (nerve sheath tumors), malignant fibrous histiocytomas, myxosarcomas, and hemangiopericytomas. Soft tissue sarcomas are locally invasive (meaning they readily invade into and through adjacent normal tissue), but they are slow to metastasize (Figures 28.1–28.4).

Soft tissue sarcomas that occur **in cats** under the skin of the neck, between the shoulder blades, the flank, and in the back leg muscles are often termed *injection site sarcomas,* or *vaccine-associated sarcomas,* due to their anatomic location at common sites for subcutaneous injection, particularly rabies and feline leukemia vaccines. The risk for a cat seems to be an individual one, rather than a high risk for all cats, but increases with more injections at the same site on the body.

## Staging

Metastasis at the time of diagnosis is uncommon; however, thoracic radiographs should be obtained as the most common site of systemic metastasis. Regional lymph nodes also should be palpated, with biopsy or aspiration cytology performed if enlarged. A CBC, serum chemistry profile and urinalysis are recommended, particularly if multiple anesthesias (such as for radiotherapy) or chemotherapy are anticipated.

The most reliable predictor of how an individual soft tissue sarcoma will behave is the **grade** of the tumor, which is determined by histopathologic examination of a biopsy. Dogs with grade 1 and 2 tumors have a high likelihood of recurrence after conservative surgery,

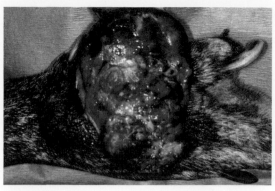

**Figure 28.1.** Soft tissue sarcomas can become ulcerated as they enlarge. This tumor is obviously painful and requires palliation. In this dog palliation would be best accomplished by amputation; however, palliative radiation could be considered as an alternative.

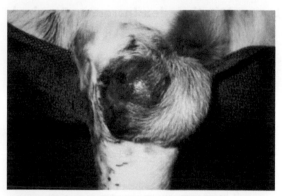

28.2

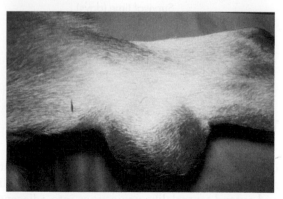

**Figure 28.2 and Figure 28.3.** When soft tissue sarcomas occur on the limbs, excision with complete margins is often impossible and other modalities are needed for tumor control. (Courtesy of Gordon H. Theilen)

28.3

but approximately 90% are tumor free 12 months after aggressive surgery. Most importantly, dogs with grade 1 and 2 tumors show very low metastatic rates (less than 15%). In addition, dogs with low mitotic index have an average survival time of 4 years. Although the overall risk of spread from a soft tissue sarcoma is low, more than 40% of dogs with grade 3 tumors show evidence of metastasis. In one study, dogs with grade 3 soft tissue sarcomas also had an average survival after surgery of only 8 months (Figure 28.5).

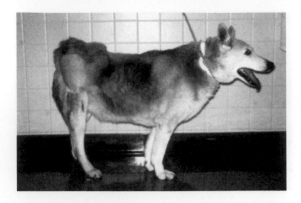

**Figure 28.4.** When soft tissue sarcomas occur on the body, complete excision is sometimes feasible, but when the tumor is very large surgery may not be anatomically possible. (Courtesy of John Berg)

## Lower Mitotic Index Increases Survival

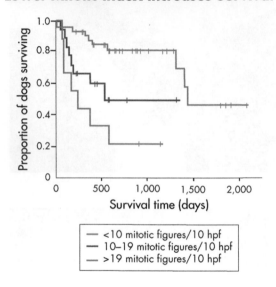

— <10 mitotic figures/10 hpf
— 10–19 mitotic figures/10 hpf
— >19 mitotic figures/10 hpf

**Figure 28.5.** Kaplan-Meier survival curve showing the effect of tumor grade on survival for dogs with soft tissue sarcomas. The effect of grade is similar for cats with this cancer type. Kuntz et al., *JAVMA* 211:1147–1151, 1997, with permission (from *Managing the Canine Cancer Patient,* Veterinary Learning Systems 2006, with permission).

## Treatment

Because they usually remain localized, treatment of grade 1 and 2 STS is primarily aimed at controlling the tumor where it occurs. Because soft tissue sarcomas are very invasive and extend tentaclelike projections into adjacent normal tissue, it is very difficult to completely remove these tumors with surgery alone. To attempt a complete excision, it is necessary to remove the tumor and a wide (usually 3 cm) margin of normal surrounding tissue, which can be difficult depending on where the tumor is on the body. The exception to this would be if the sarcoma occurs on an extremity such as a limb, where amputation can be performed. Regardless, the best chance of achieving a surgical cure for soft tissue sarcoma is with an aggressive approach at the first surgery, and repeated attempts at excision are rarely successful.

A combination of both surgery and high doses of radiation therapy provides the best chance of controlling otherwise inoperable tumors.

Chemotherapy given after surgery has the greatest chance of slowing down or preventing metastases, and is recommended for dogs with grade 3 sarcomas. It is important to remember that even for dogs with grade 3 tumors, 60% of patients do not develop metastasis, so treatment of the primary tumor is still a priority.

## Nursing Highlights

Postoperative pain relief is the most important aspect of treatment for dogs with soft tissue sarcoma. For wide surgical resections, when there is tension on the wound edges, firm, comfortable bandages will assist in healing, protect the surgery site from licking and chewing, and enable better pain relief.

## Case Example

Buddy, an 11-year-old, castrated male, 45 kg German shepherd, had a soft tissue mass noticed on the dorsal surface of the left carpus 12 months previously, and it was debulked at that time; a regrowth was again debulked 8 months later, and at the most recent presentation, it was a $6 \times 5 \times 3$ cm mass that was not ulcerated and did not radiographically involve the underlying bone. Histopathology of an incisional biopsy yielded a diagnosis of a soft tissue sarcoma. The cells were moderately pleomorphic and the mitotic index was given as <10 per 10 hpf; patchy necrosis was reported so this was a grade 2 STS. Thoracic radiographs showed no evidence of metastasis. The regional lymph nodes were not palpable due to obesity. A preanesthetic screen showed azotemia, which may have been prerenal, but urine specific gravity, while not isosthenuric, was not adequately concentrated (1.025) if he was dehydrated. Buddy was not reported to have any other clinical symptoms related to the tumor or other problems.

### Further Staging

The external regional lymph nodes (prescapular and axillary) should be identified by ultrasonography and biopsy or aspiration cytology performed if enlarged.

A CBC, and repeat chemistry panel and urinalysis (with culture, to rule out pyelonephritis) are recommended due to the azotemia, particularly if multiple anesthesias (such as for radiotherapy) or chemotherapy is anticipated.

### Case Resolution

Repeated blood work showed resolution of the azotemia, and amputation was recommended as the most likely treatment to result in a cure. Buddy's owners declined amputation; and debulking surgery and radiotherapy was performed (54 Gray total dose in daily 3 Gy fractions, 5 days a week). He developed postradiation moist desquamation that was managed with topical cleaning and NSAIDs until it healed 2 weeks after radiation. Two years after radiotherapy he was alive and well, with no evidence of tumor recurrence.

# Splenic Hemangiosarcoma in Dogs

## 29

## Overview

Hemangiosarcoma is the most common malignant tumor of the spleen in dogs. The tumor in the spleen (Figure 29.1) causes dogs to feel ill, and it is very dangerous because it can rupture and cause sudden and severe internal bleeding. Hemangiosarcoma also has a very high propensity to metastasize, particularly to the liver. The surgical removal of the spleen alleviates the primary symptoms and the immediate risk of sudden internal bleeding; however, almost all dogs with splenic hemangiosarcoma will eventually develop metastasis.

## Staging

The expected survival time for dogs with hemangiosarcoma after surgery depends on the ability of additional treatment, usually chemotherapy, to delay the development of metastasis. This is largely related to the clinical stage of the tumor in the spleen. Stage 1 tumors are confined to the spleen with no evidence of metastasis, whereas dogs with stage 2 disease have a ruptured spleen, with or without regional lymph node involvement. Stage 3 tumors are large, invasive tumors with distant metastases. Staging therefore should include abdominal ultrasonography (Figure 29.2) (often supplemented by the surgery report) and thoracic radiographs; a CBC, serum chemistry profile, and urinalysis will help ensure that the dog is otherwise healthy. Up to 25% of dogs with splenic hemangiosarcoma may also have a right atrial hemangiosarcoma; ideally, therefore, it is important to examine the right atrial appendage by ultrasonography for presence of a mass prior to making firm recommendations for adjunctive therapy.

There may also be some predictive value to the histologic grade of the tumor, a score assigned by the pathologist based on the tumor's histologic appearance.

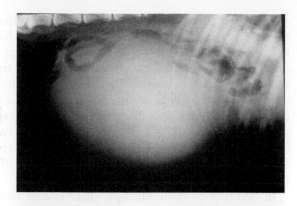

**Figure 29.1.** Hemangiosarcoma often presents with a dog that is feeling unwell, with a distended abdomen. Here, radiographs disclose a large cranioventral abdominal mass. The location is suggestive of a splenic mass. Histopathology is necessary to make a diagnosis of hemangiosarcoma, however. (Courtesy of John Berg)

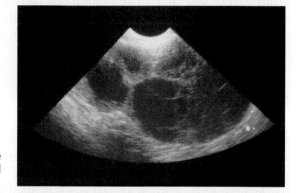

**Figure 29.2.** Abdominal ultrasonography of the same dog in Figure 29.1 shows a large, cavitated splenic mass. (Courtesy of John Berg)

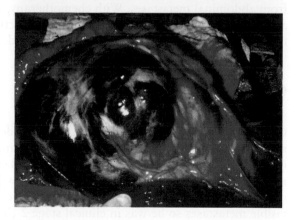

**Figure 29.3.** At exploratory laparotomy of the same dog in Figures 29.1 and 29.2, the large splenic mass is found to be intact. It is important to examine the rest of the abdomen. (Courtesy of John Berg)

## Treatment

Splenectomy (Figure 29.3) is the definitive treatment for this disease. Improvement in symptoms is usually rapid and quality of life is improved. In addition, the short-term risk of internal bleeding is reduced. However, when metastasis is present, additional treatment is needed to attempt to extend survival time. With surgery alone, dogs with stage 1 tumors have an average survival of 12 months, compared to 3 to 5 months for dogs with stage 2 hemangiosarcoma and 2 months for dogs with stage 3 tumors.

The good effect of chemotherapy on some other cancers in dogs raised hopes that drug therapy may also improve survival for dogs with hemangiosarcoma. However, the response has been less successful with this disease. For dogs with stage 1 or 2 disease, chemotherapy does appear to approximately double survival times over surgery alone. For dogs with stage 3 tumors, the benefit of chemotherapy is less clear.

In one study of dogs with metastasis treated with surgery and chemotherapy together, dogs in which all the visible cancer both in the spleen and elsewhere could be removed, survived an average of 6 months; dogs whose cancer could not be completely removed lived an average of 2 months. The chemotherapy medication most likely to provide a response in hemangiosarcoma is doxorubicin, and other medications may also have a role to play in the treatment of this difficult disease.

In addition to chemotherapy, there is also some possibility that antiangiogenic treatments—treatment targeted at tumor blood vessels—may slow the growth of hemangiosarcoma metastases. However, this is experimental and chemotherapy is more likely to be effective. Many veterinary oncologists suggest an antiangiogenic approach **in combination** with chemotherapy.

## Nursing Highlights

Most dogs do very well postoperatively and with the exception of pain control, do not require supportive care—at least initially. In later stages of disease, they may require analgesics, antiinflammatories, appetite stimulants, and corticosteroids. Blood transfusions (packed red cells or whole blood) could be used judiciously as needed if bleeding occurs from abdominal metastases. With chemotherapy, supportive care could include antibiotics and appetite stimulants when needed. Prophylactic trimethoprim-sulpha for 14 days each time doxorubicin is given reduces the risk of side effects from that drug.

## Case Example

Conner, a 7-year-old, castrated male, 35 kg golden retriever had a history of hemoabdomen. Abdominal ultrasonography revealed a 5 cm splenic mass but no other visible lesions in other abdominal organs. A hemangiosarcoma of the spleen was diagnosed after splenectomy, and based on the pathology report it was a grade 3 tumor. At surgery there was no gross evidence of mesenteric seeding, and liver and regional lymph nodes did not have visible metastases so he was in clinical stage 2 (because it was ruptured). Thoracic radiographs were reported to show no detectable metastases or abnormal heart base. Postoperatively his PCV rose to over 40%. A preoperative serum chemistry profile and urinalysis were normal.

### Further Staging

If further treatment is anticipated, a pretreatment (postoperative) abdominal ultrasonogram will provide a baseline for future assessments of efficacy. Examine also the right atrial appendage by ultrasonography.

A careful physical examination of his cardiovascular system should be done, and baseline cardiac ultrasonography can be evaluated when the atrium is examined. If ultrasonography shows any evidence at all of ventricular dilation or reduced shortening fraction, doxorubicin is contraindicated.

## Case Resolution

The best chance to improve Conner's survival time was felt to be adjunctive chemotherapy. Cardiac ultrasonography showed no evidence of a heart base mass, but Conner's cardiac function (specifically his fractional shortening) was abnormal and low. For this reason, doxorubicin was not considered to be a good choice for therapy (due to concerns about exacerbating his cardiac muscle damage), and mitoxantrone was substituted in a combination chemotherapy protocol. Conner completed his chemotherapy, and at a recheck ultrasonogram, his abdomen showed no evidence of metastasis. Unfortunately, about 4 months after completing chemotherapy (8 months from splenectomy) he again collapsed and multiple bleeding hepatic metastases were identified on ultrasonography. His owner elected no further chemotherapy, but he responded to blood transfusion and antiinflammatories and regained approximately 80% of his strength and exercise abilities. A further 2 weeks later he again collapsed and his owner elected euthanasia.

# Osteosarcoma in Dogs

30

## Overview

Osteosarcoma, a malignant tumor arising in bone, is one of the most common cancers of dogs. The tumor affects primarily large breeds of dogs, often at relatively young ages. The cause is unknown. Although osteosarcoma is a serious disease, with treatment, the vast majority of dogs can be significantly helped.

Osteosarcoma behaves in a fairly predictable fashion. The tumor in the leg is very painful, because small fractures and bleeding cause pressure on the sensitive nerve endings in the surface of the affected bone (Figure 30.1). Occasionally, the leg may fracture (see Chapter 23) completely, which necessitates immediate treatment. Osteosarcoma almost always metastasizes to the lungs prior to diagnosis, although at the time of diagnosis, the lung tumors are usually microscopic and cannot be seen on thoracic radiographs. In treating the disease, we must treat the tumor in both the leg and the lungs.

## Staging

In addition to radiographs of the affected leg (Figure 30.2), thoracic radiographs, regional lymph node evaluation, and CBC, serum biochemistry profile and urinalysis are recommended **prior to surgery**.

Dogs that have pulmonary metastases that are radiographically detectable at the time of presentation have a poor prognosis.

Dogs with **preamputation** elevations (as measured on a serum chemistry profile) of serum alkaline phosphatase (ALP) tend to have more aggressive osteosarcomas. Although serum ALP does not absolutely determine the chance of long-term survival, it has a great impact on reducing the chances of response to chemotherapy (Figure 30.3).

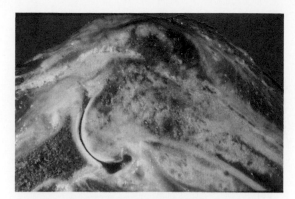

**Figure 30.1.** A sectioned specimen of an osteosarcoma shows cortical disruption, periosteal new bone production, and a mild pathologic fracture in the proximal humerus.

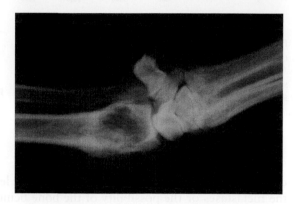

**Figure 30.2.** A radiograph of an osteosarcoma of the distal radius showing marked lysis of the bone surrounded by periosteal new bone production. Note that the lesion does not cross the joint space (all changes restricted to the radius), which is a strong indicator of cancer in this location.

Another very important prognostic factor identified for dogs with appendicular osteosarcoma is the histologic grade. Dogs are more likely to have grade 3 tumors, however those with low-grade tumors have a better prognosis even with less aggressive treatment. In addition, mitotic index is a predictor of survival with increasing numbers of mitoses correlating with a poor prognosis.

Finally, dogs that have evidence of metastasis to the regional lymph node have a shorter median survival (2 months) than if no metastasis are found (10.5 months), mirroring the poor prognosis if thoracic metastases are visible at diagnosis.

## Treatment

For the majority of dogs, amputation is the best treatment for the tumor in the leg. Amputation is performed primarily to alleviate the pain produced by the tumor, and also to prevent the leg being broken (Figure 30.4). Amputation is discussed in more detail in Chapter 6.

Life expectancy following surgery alone is limited, because the lung metastases continue to grow. On the average, dogs live 5 months after surgery, and approximately 10% of dogs live over 1 year. Nevertheless, we still recommend amputation as the best method of relieving pain and maximizing quality of life during the survival time. Pain relief allows considerable improvement in the patient's quality of life. A second, but less effective, option for dogs that cannot be treated by amputation is radiotherapy for pain relief. This proce-

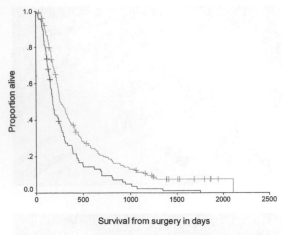

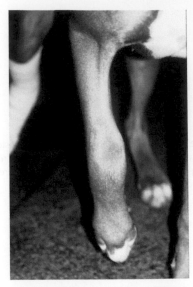

**Figure 30.3.** A Kaplan-Meier survival curve showing the effect of high serum ALP level (red line) and normal serum ALP (green line) prior to amputation and chemotherapy on survival of dogs with osteosarcoma. Dogs with a normal serum ALP lived longer on average. Moore et al., *J Vet Internal Med* 21:783–790, 2007, with permission.

**Figure 30.4.** A painful swollen distal leg in a boxer with osteosarcoma of the distal radius.

dure allows approximately 80% of dogs to feel less pain, but does not prevent growth of the metastases or the possibility of the bone being broken.

Because amputation does not prevent growth of the metastases, the most important advance in treatment of osteosarcoma has been the finding that chemotherapy following surgery can slow the growth of the metastases, dramatically improve life expectancy, and in some cases result in a cure. Past experience has shown that three chemotherapeutic medications—cisplatin, carboplatin, and doxorubicin—are effective in treating dogs with osteosarcoma. Overall (not accounting for elevations in ALP), approximately 45% of dogs live over 1 year when either of these drugs is given alone, and many dogs live much longer. The final choice of drug is often influenced by factors other than the tumor; for example, a Doberman would not be a good candidate for doxorubicin due to higher risk of cardiotoxicity in that breed. Many oncologists recommend, for dogs that are otherwise healthy, a chemotherapy protocol that combines doxorubicin and carboplatin. For dogs completing this protocol without developing metastases, the overall chances of living 2 years beyond amputation are about 25%, and approximately 20% of dogs live 3 years or their normal lifespan.

## Nursing Highlights

Pain relief (see also Chapter 11) is the most important aspect of treatment for dogs with osteosarcoma, either while they are waiting for surgery, or if their owner refuses amputation. Bone pain is notoriously refractory to medical management, but with multimodality pain relief, comfort levels can be improved. In addition, changes to their environment (ramps, etc.) will assist the patient's comfort level (see also Chapter 11).

In brief, nonsteroidal antiinflammatories (NSAIDs) can be helpful, but they usually do not control the pain themselves. Options include piroxicam, carprofen, or metacam, but these cannot be combined with each other. Corticosteroids are not usually particularly helpful, but they can be tried; however, they must not be combined with NSAIDs. Tramadol can be combined with NSAIDs and opioids to reduce the effective dosage of all drugs. Narcotics can also be combined with NSAIDs. When instituting a new narcotic therapy, the nurse might encounter a possibility of patient sedation; this usually will pass in the first few days of treatment.

We find codeine particularly helpful for "breakthrough" pain at nighttime and fentanyl patches may give more consistent pain relief, but care should be exercised in houses where other pets or children could ingest a patch lost from the patient. If a fentanyl patch is used, it can take 24 hours for blood levels to rise so dogs can be given a "loading dose" of injectable fentanyl IV.

Aminobisphosphonates inhibit osteoclast activity and so can reduce osteolysis and the resultant pain and fracture risk. The response is slow, though, and it can take up to 2 weeks for pain relief to become apparent. Care should be taken with orally administered bisphosphonates because esophageal irritation can occur particularly in patients that lie down after taking the drug. See Chapter 11 for details as to how to avoid this risk.

## Case Example

Rani, a 5-year-old spayed female, 32 kg, Borzoi had a non–weight-bearing left hindlimb lameness; radiographs showed a lytic and productive lesion of the proximal tibia. The popliteal lymph node was not enlarged. Thoracic radiographs showed no evidence of pulmonary metastases. CBC and serum chemistry profile were normal, including the serum ALP level, which is an important positive prognostic factor. Amputation biopsy confirmed the lesion to be a high-grade osteosarcoma (high mitotic index [54 per 10 hpf], necrosis, and pleomorphism).

### Case Resolution

Amputation was performed and Rani recovered well. Chemotherapy was recommended, but there was concern that her risk of cardiac toxicity was moderate if doxorubicin was given, due to a possible breed (Borzoi) predisposition to cardiomyopathy. In one study of over 300 dogs with osteosarcoma treated with doxorubicin, one of the 3 Borzois entered developed clinical cardiomyopathy. This rate was higher than for dogs of most other breeds, but obviously it was a small number of dogs. The availability of alternative chemotherapy drugs with similar efficacy (carboplatin and cisplatin) suggests that doxorubicin was not the first choice for adjunctive treatment of osteosarcoma in Rani. She therefore received a protocol of carboplatin alone. She was still free of detectable metastases 2 years later, although she required nonsteroidal antiinflammatories due to worsening joint discomfort in her other legs.

# Oral Melanoma in Dogs

## 31

## Overview

Tumors of the oral cavity are fairly common in older dogs. Unfortunately, they are usually malignant, with both local infiltration and metastasis presenting significant problems. Symptoms usually relate to the primary tumor impinging on the dog's ability to eat comfortably. Oral melanomas are friable and invasive within the soft tissues of the mouth, often causing bleeding (Figures 31.1 and 31.2). Without any treatment, survival time is usually only a few months because of the progression of these symptoms.

Metastasis of tumors is probably an early event; however, metastases are often not detected until some time after the primary melanoma is resected. The growth rate of metastases may vary, but once lymph node metastasis is found, the chances for long survival reduce (average survival less than 6 months) and chemotherapy becomes important in treatment strategies. If metastasis to the lungs is seen, unless there is a good response to treatment, survival time is usually less than 4 months.

Studies in dogs without obvious metastases have found that the size of the tumor may predict survival after treatment, with significantly longer survival for dogs with small (<2 cm diameter) tumors (average = 17 months) than for dogs with larger tumors (average = 5.4 months) (Figure 31.3). Studies have also indicated that dogs with tumors in the front of the lower jaw, the back cheek, or the lip seem to have longer remissions and survival after surgery. Another study found longer survival times for dogs with tumors that had low numbers of mitotic figures on biopsy. A combination of all of these factors is probably the most powerful predictor of survival.

## Staging

Prior to starting treatment, thoracic radiographs should be examined for metastases to the lungs and to make sure the lungs and heart appear healthy otherwise. Lymph nodes should

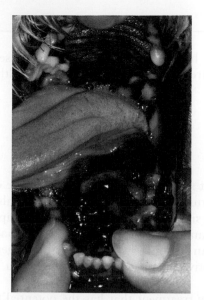

**Figure 31.1.** Melanoma is the most common tumor in the mouth of dogs. Even though it is a highly metastatic tumor, the quality of life impact of the primary tumor in the mouth is the most life-threatening aspect of the disease for most dogs.

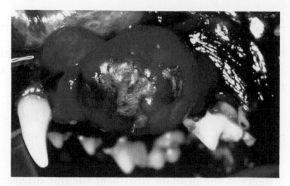

**Figure 31.2.** Although melanoma usually has the characteristic heavily pigmented appearance, it is not always pigmented and must still be considered as a diagnostic differential for nonpigmented tumors.

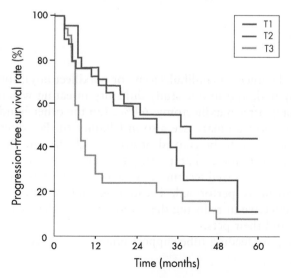

**Dogs with Smaller Oral Tumors of Any Type Live Longer**

**Figure 31.3.** Kaplan-Meier survival curve showing the effect of tumor size, for any type of oral tumor, on survival after treatment with surgery and radiation therapy. Theon et al., *JAVMA* 210:778–784, 1997, with permission (from *Managing the Canine Cancer Patient*, Veterinary Learning Systems 2006, with permission).

be examined by palpation, cytology, and possibly biopsy for presence of metastases. Finally, routine blood work should be done to ensure that the dog is otherwise healthy before proceeding with chemotherapy.

## Treatment

Surgery is the primary treatment for this disease, but surgical cure is difficult, because of both the anatomy of the area and the infiltrative nature of the tumors. Surgery may also help to improve the success of other treatment types, such as radiation and chemotherapy.

Radiotherapy has been reported for this disease, and when available may allow long-term control of the cancer even when surgery is not an option, or as an adjunct to surgery and chemotherapy. Radiotherapy may also be palliative for dogs with oral melanoma in later stages of cancer growth.

When metastasis occurs, chemotherapy is the only treatment that has the potential to extend survival for this disease; the best chemotherapy medications known for this tumor are carboplatin and other platinum drugs.

Radiotherapy and chemotherapy combined have given the best survival rates for dogs where surgery is not complete. In one study of dogs treated with this combination, only 15% had local recurrence, usually within the first 5 months, and about half the dogs developed metastatic disease within an average time of 10 months. Average survival time for all treated dogs was 1 year. Without surgery or radiation therapy, about 30% of dogs will respond to chemotherapy for a period of around 6 months. Even with this treatment, cure is often not possible, but survival time can often be increased.

## Nursing Highlights

Following extensive oral surgery (mandibulectomy or maxillectomy), some problems with eating would be anticipated, and in one study difficulty in eating was noted for 44% of the dogs (most commonly after maxillectomy; 64%). On the other hand, pain was felt to be less after surgery for most animals (see also in Chapter 6). Postoperative analgesia is important, and dogs may need to be coaxed or even taught to eat. During this time the nurse can help owners identify foods that are easy to prehend and swallow, and may even be able to demonstrate hand-assisted feeding techniques. Antibiotics are important regardless of whether treatment is performed, because secondary infections are common. Metronidazole is very effective in reducing the severe halitosis that may interfere with the bond between owners and their pets.

Most dogs do not require feeding tube support unless surgery is extensive or radiation side effects are severe.

## Case Example

Bindi, an 8-year-old, spayed female, 10.2 kg, Maltese-cross had a 1 cm melanoma of the oral lip/skin margin in a rostral location that was excised for biopsy. The original biopsy showed narrow, but complete, margins. Further, more aggressive, surgery was performed, and margins were assessed as adequate on repeated histopathology. Histopathology on the original tumor described a mitotic rate of more than 1 per high power field (>10 per 10 hpf). Lymph nodes were normal in size, and thoracic radiographs showed no evidence of metastases. CBC, serum chemistry profile, and urinalysis showed no evidence of metabolic disease.

Since Bindi had a stage 1 tumor of the lip, the only possibly negative prognostic factor was the mitotic rate of >10 per 10 high power fields, which is borderline high.

## Case Resolution

The best primary treatment for Bindi was considered to be an aggressive surgery, which had already been done. Since Bindi was otherwise well, and her mitotic rate was borderline high, adjunctive carboplatin chemotherapy was also recommended; chemotherapy is always more likely to be successful when there is minimal residual disease. On the other hand, her prognosis was considered to be good even with local treatment alone. If a patient like Bindi survives a long time after chemotherapy, you can never be sure she wasn't going to anyway! In this situation the dilemma is best posed as follows: If the question is, "Can we get by without chemotherapy?" then the answer is yes, Bindi may be okay without it although there is a risk. Whereas if the client's approach is, "I want to do the best thing to ensure that Bindi's chances of remaining disease-free are maximized" then the answer is, chemotherapy will improve her chances.

Bindi did not receive chemotherapy, and 16 months after surgery, lymph node metastasis was detected and pulmonary metastases were confirmed. Her owners declined further definitive therapy and opted for palliation.

# Oral Squamous Cell Carcinoma in Cats

## Overview

The most common mouth cancer in cats is squamous cell carcinoma (SCC). They arise from the mucosal lining of the mouth, commonly under the tongue (Figure 32.1) or around the teeth (Figure 32.2), and are friable and invasive, often causing bleeding and pain. Unfortunately they are malignant, with infiltration into surrounding structures in the mouth presenting the most significant problem. Symptoms usually relate to the primary tumor impinging on the cat's ability to eat comfortably. They can invade into underlying bone, but rarely spread to distant sites in the body. About 20% will spread to the lymph nodes nearby; these are usually larger tumors located toward the back of the mouth. Because these tumors are often advanced, survival time is usually only a few weeks without any treatment because of the progression of these symptoms.

Oral SCC is associated with tobacco use in human patients, and a weak association with exposure to environmental tobacco smoke has also been made in cats. In addition, cats that wear a flea collar have 5 times the risk of oral SCC as cats that do not, and cats with high canned food intake had a 3 times the risk of developing oral SCC. It is possible that poor oral hygiene plays a role in pathogenesis as it does in humans.

## Staging

Particularly because these cats are often older and medically unstable, some testing is needed to determine the extent of the cancer and to evaluate them for other diseases that could impact prognosis or response to therapy. This generally involves CBC and serum chemistry profile, serum T4, urinalysis, radiographs, and careful evaluation of the lymph nodes. The finding of metastasis to either the lymph nodes or lungs denotes a poor

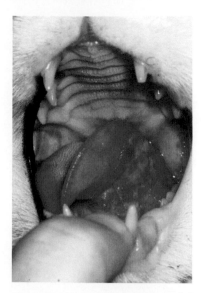

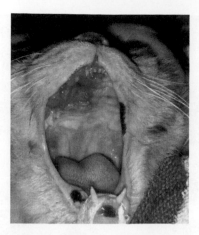

**Figure 32.2.** Another common location for oral squamous cell carcinoma in cats is around the teeth. This is a notoriously difficult tumor to control with treatment.

**Figure 32.1.** Squamous cell carcinoma is the most common tumor in the mouth of older cats. A classic location is under the tongue. Although the tumor has a very low metastatic rate, the quality of life impact of the primary tumor in the mouth is huge and these cats unfortunately have short survival time.

prognosis. For very large or erosive cancers a CT scan or MRI may help determine the depth of the cancer.

## Treatment

Surgery is the primary treatment for this disease in dogs and people, but in cats it rarely improves symptoms or survival times unless the tumor is very small (Figures 32.3 and 32.4). Average survival times for cats treated by surgery alone are less than 2 months.

Radiotherapy has been reported for this disease, and may be palliative for pain, but again it rarely causes significant improvement in survival times. Average survival times for cats treated by radiotherapy alone are 3 to 4 months.

Chemotherapy for this disease is rarely warranted, because the risk of metastasis is low, but it is the only treatment that has the potential to extend survival when metastases are seen. The best chemotherapy medications known for this tumor are doxorubicin and carboplatin. One problem with these drugs is that safe administration requires good kidney function, and often the older cats affected with SCC have underlying kidney disease.

The NSAID piroxicam may provide some symptomatic relief, but it rarely causes tumor shrinkage. One study showed longer survival times when this medication was used, but still average survival was less than 4 months.

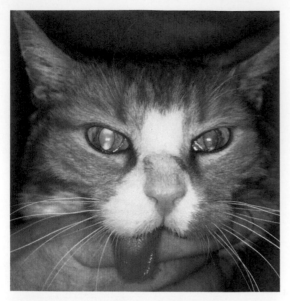

32.3

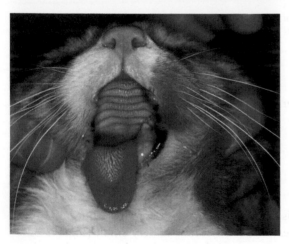

32.4

**Figure 32.3 and Figure 32.4.** Although the prognosis for most cats with oral squamous cell carcinoma is poor, when the tumor is diagnosed early, aggressive local treatment may occasionally be successful. This cat recovered well from an aggressive bilateral mandibulectomy and had a good quality of life, with dramatically extended survival time (more than 1 year, which is when the photographs were taken).

## Nursing Highlights

Supportive care is possibly the most important aspect of treatment in this often older, delicate group of patients. We have seen significant improvement in overall wellbeing and quality of life in cats treated with only a feeding tube for nutritional support, in conjunction with pain relief. In addition, management of any other problems such as renal or heart disease is important in this older group of patients.

## Case Example

Billie, a 14-year-old, FS DSH, 5 kg was noticed by her owner to be drooling and favoring softer foods; on examination a large erosive tumor was found associated with her left mandible from the symphysis to the first premolar. Biopsy showed this to be an oral SCC with a high mitotic rate. Routine blood work was reported to be normal, but a urinalysis was not evaluated. Surgical resection was attempted, but it was incomplete. The mandibular node on that side was enlarged and was biopsied at surgery, showing evidence of metastasis to the node.

## *Case Resolution*

After surgery Billie was eating well and polydypsic. Chemotherapy was planned to start 2 weeks after surgery, but during this period, her appetite reduced and she began to lose weight. Reevaluation of her blood work showed her to be azotemic, and her urine specific gravity was isosthenuric. Chemotherapy was delayed while supportive care was instituted for her renal failure, but her condition deteriorated and she was euthanatized. This case serves to emphasize the importance of complete evaluation of older patients with cancer; particularly if aggressive treatment strategies are being considered.

# Mammary Carcinoma in Dogs

## Overview

Mammary (breast) tumors account for almost half of all cancers seen in female dogs. Intact females have a sevenfold increased risk of developing mammary cancer compared to neutered females, and studies clearly indicate the preventive role of spaying **prior to the second heat.**

## Staging

Although most (75%) mammary tumors are either benign, or if malignant, have not metastasized, approximately 25% have metastasized by the lymphatics or the bloodstream at the time of diagnosis. The two most common sites of metastasis are the lymph nodes closest to the tumor (regional lymph nodes) (Figure 33.1) and the lungs (Figure 33.2). Therefore, evaluation of a pet with mammary cancer will include thoracic radiographs, full blood work and urinalysis, and careful evaluation of regional lymph nodes by palpation, and (if enlarged or firm) biopsy.

### Prognostic Factors

Tumor size is one of the most important prognostic factors for a dog with a mammary mass. Dogs with mammary tumors less than 3 cm in diameter have a much higher likelihood of being cured by treatment than dogs with larger tumors (Figures 33.3 and 33.4).

Metastasis to regional lymph nodes has been associated with an increased risk for tumor recurrence and for decreased overall survival after surgery.

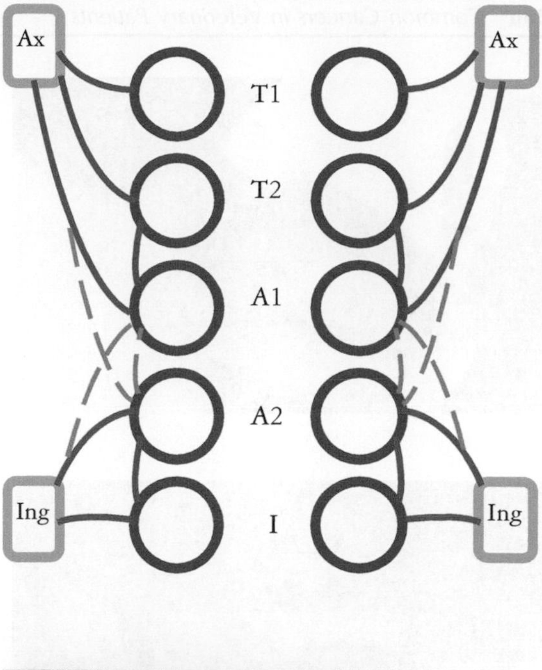

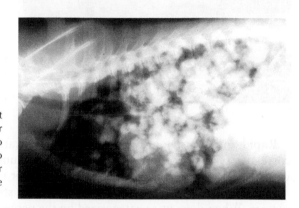

**Figure 33.1.** A schematic showing the lymphatic draining of the canine mammary glands. Note that there is some cross-drainage, so it is important to carefully palpate all the mammary glands and lymph nodes in dogs with a mammary gland tumor.
T = thoracic
A = abdominal
I = inguinal
Ax = axillary lymph node
Ing = inguinal lymph node

**Figure 33.2.** The lungs are one of the most common locations for mammary gland tumor metastasis. When taking thoracic radiographs to screen for pulmonary metastases, it is important to take both lateral views as well as a dorsoventral or ventrodorsal view, because some lesions are visible on one lateral but not the other.

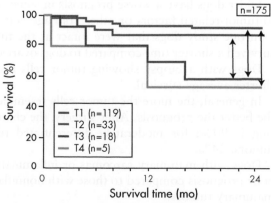

**Figure 33.3.** Kaplan-Meier survival curve showing the effect of tumor size of survival after surgery for dogs with mammary cancer. Those with smaller tumors live longer on average. Yamagami et al., *J Vet Med Sci* 58:1079–1083, 1996, with permission (from *Managing the Canine Cancer Patient*, Veterinary Learning Systems 2006, with permission).

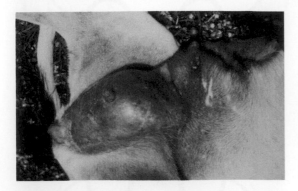

**Figure 33.4.** Tumor diameter is one of the most important prognostic factors for dogs with mammary gland tumors. This dog with a large tumor will unfortunately have a poor prognosis; if the tumor had been addressed earlier, it could have been quite treatable, underscoring the need to remind dog owners to be vigilant in screening intact female dogs for mammary masses and have them treated when small.

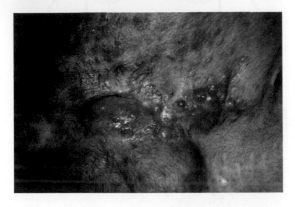

**Figure 33.5.** Inflammatory mammary carcinoma is an extremely painful invasive form of mammary carcinoma. These dogs have a poor prognosis and require a great deal of supportive care.

Rapid and invasive growth, often seen as fixation of the tumor to the overlying skin, correlates with a worse prognosis. Dogs with tumors that ulcerate overlying skin have a worse prognosis than dogs with tumors without ulceration.

Diet and body weight were important in one study for dogs with malignant mammary tumors. When dogs were categorized by the percent of total calories they derived from fat and protein, the average survival time after surgery for dogs fed a low fat diet (<39%) with protein greater than 27%, 23–27%, and less than 23% was 3 years, 1.2 years, and 6 months, respectively. Dogs that have a mammary carcinoma may benefit from a low fat, high protein diet after surgery.

Older dogs have a worse prognosis in some studies but it is unclear whether this is due to tumor-related factors or other "old age" diseases.

In one study dogs that were intact at the time of surgery for a mammary carcinoma survived a shorter time compared to dogs ovariectomised within the 2 years before surgery.

Dogs with a biopsy showing tumor cells invading blood or lymphatic vessels have a shorter average survival.

In general, the more the tumor cells resemble normal breast cells (well differentiated), the better the prognosis. After surgery, the chance of a poorly differentiated tumor recurring is 90%; for moderately differentiated tumors, 68%; and for well-differentiated tumors, 24%.

Dogs with mammary sarcomas or inflammatory carcinomas (Figure 33.5) have a very poor prognosis compared to those with noninflammatory carcinomas or mixed malignant mammary tumors.

Complete removal of the tumor as assessed by histopathology has been shown to increase the length of survival.

## Treatment

The surgery plan needs to be extensive enough to remove all cancer tissue. This may mean that a second surgery may need to be performed when the borders around a mammary cancer are narrow. Radiation therapy, as used in human breast cancer patients, may also decrease the risk of recurrence where complete surgery is not possible. For dogs with mammary tumors that have one or more poor prognostic factors listed above, systemic chemotherapy is the most likely to improve their chances of remission and survival.

## Nursing Highlights

Since size of the tumor is important in prognosis after treatment, all adult female dogs, particularly those that are intact, or those that have already had a tumor removed, should have their mammary glands palpated thoroughly at regular intervals in order to detect tumors at the earliest time possible. Caregivers should be instructed in a proper technique for examination.

To reduce the risk of mammary carcinoma, clients should be counseled to ovariectomize their dogs before the first estrus, and to ensure that weight control is practiced in at least the first year of life. Because one study showed dogs with a higher intake of red meat in their diet were also at higher risk for developing mammary cancer, it may be better to feed a commercial food that ensures that calories are primarily from other sources.

Nutritional support, and possibly diet modifications as suggested above under prognostic factors, could be important for dogs with mammary carcinomas. Pain relief after surgery, particularly if the surgery is extensive, is mandatory. Inflammatory carcinomas have a major impact on quality of life, and supportive care is extremely important in this group of dogs, using antiinflammatories, analgesics, and antibiotics.

## Case Example

Reba, a 10-year-old, female, 21 kg, Airedale terrier had a 1 cm axillary mass that grew to approximately 3 cm in diameter over 6 months. First excision resulted in histologically incomplete margins. After scar revision (second) surgery, the mass was completely excised, but metastasis was present in the axillary lymph node. She had not been spayed. Thoracic radiographs revealed no evidence of metastases. Preanesthetic serum chemistry profile showed no abnormalities. Reba also had dilated cardiomyopathy (marginally low fractional shortening) and was receiving treatment for that condition.

## Further Staging

A CBC and urinalysis (with culture, if indicated) are recommended before starting chemotherapy.

It is useful to repeat 3-view thoracic radiographs periodically (every 3 months in the absence of clinical problems) to monitor for the development of pulmonary metastases.

Because of the lymph node metastasis, Reba was considered to be in stage 4 (of 5) mammary carcinoma. Based on the literature, dogs in stage 4 have a median survival time **with surgery alone** of 3 months and 13% were alive 1 year after surgery, so chemotherapy was recommended.

## Case Resolution

Due to her cardiac condition, doxorubicin was contraindicated. Therefore the recommended course of treatment for Reba was chemotherapy consisting of mitoxantrone in combination with carboplatin and piroxicam. The chances for a cure were considered to be low, but the expected median survival was 9–12 months. Reba completed her protocol with no toxicity except for neutropenia after the first mitoxantrone that necessitated a dose reduction of 25% for all subsequent treatments of that drug. Fourteen months after surgery she was still clear of metastases at examination and thoracic radiographs. Her cardiac function had deteriorated, and she was referred to a cardiologist for further evaluation.

# Mammary Carcinoma in Cats

## Overview

Tumors of the mammary glands in cats are most often carcinomas; benign tumors and other types of malignant tumors are rare. Mammary carcinomas are seen in older cats, especially if intact. Tri-colored and Siamese cats are at increased risk for developing mammary cancer. DSH and younger cats tend to do better with this disease.

Mammary carcinomas in cats may remain undetected until they become quite large or ulcerative (Figure 34.1). Thus, unfortunately, mammary carcinoma is often advanced by the time a veterinarian is consulted. Multiple gland involvement may be seen, and in some cats the entire mammary chain is affected. Cats with tumors smaller than 3 cm diameter have both longer remissions after surgery and longer survival times.

## Staging

Feline mammary carcinoma is an invasive and often rapidly spreading tumor. It can metastasize to both the lungs and the lymph nodes. Some testing is needed to determine the extent of the cancer. This involves blood work, urinalysis, radiographs, and careful evaluation of the lymph nodes. The finding of metastasis to either the lymph nodes or lungs denotes a poor prognosis after surgery. Staging takes into account the tumor size and presence of any metastases and is useful in predicting the likely prognosis of an individual cat with this disease. Cats with small tumors and no metastases have an average survival time of nearly 30 months after surgical removal. Likewise, a histologic grading scheme (assigned by the pathologist based on the microscopic appearance of the tumor) also has predictive value. Cats with inflammatory mammary carcinomas have a worse prognosis and also require extra supportive care including analgesia because their tumors are typically very painful (Figure 34.2).

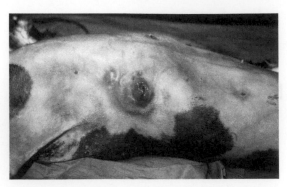

**Figure 34.1.**   This large ulcerated mammary tumor on a cat should be removed with the widest possible margins. In addition, draining lymph nodes should be biopsied at the time of surgery. (Courtesy of Dr. Gregory Ogilvie)

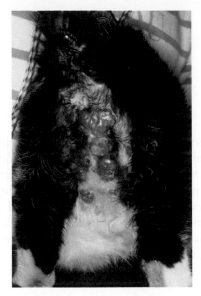

**Figure 34.2.**   This cat with multiple ulcerated inflammatory mammary carcinomas in the inguinal region requires extra supportive care, especially analgesia.

## Treatment

Feline mammary carcinomas need to be treated aggressively (Figure 34.3). Surgery alone is unlikely to provide a cure unless the tumor is very small and localized; however, even in cats with larger tumors, it does play a role in reducing local recurrence and improving survival time.

Due to the high metastatic potential of mammary carcinoma, chemotherapy appears to be the most likely treatment modality to improve survival as an adjuvant to surgery. However, few studies have reported the use of chemotherapy. At the present time, doxorubicin and possibly carboplatin appear to be the adjuvant chemotherapy drugs of choice.

Radiation therapy has been used in some cats for the treatment of mammary carcinoma and may be effective in helping to prevent local recurrence after surgery. It may also be

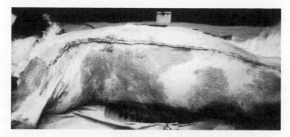

**Figure 34.3.** Cats presented with a mammary tumor should always undergo full physical examination, and all other mammary glands as well as all lymph nodes should be palpated. Mammary tumors may be multiple, and when this occurs the best surgical approach is often a full-chain mastectomy. Cats that have undergone full-chain mastectomy require supportive care, especially analgesia. (Courtesy of Dr. Gregory Ogilvie)

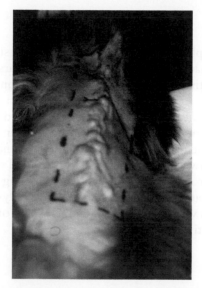

**Figure 34.4.** This cat has experienced multiple local tumor recurrence along the suture line. She is being prepared for palliative radiation therapy to attempt to reduce the tumor size and make her more comfortable.

used in some cases to try to reduce inoperable tumors so that they can be removed. Finally, radiation may be used toward to the end of a cat's life to reduce the discomfort associated with mammary carcinoma (termed *palliative radiation*) (Figure 34.4).

## Nursing Highlights

Analgesia is used during and after surgical removal of any mammary tumor, particularly when a full-chain mastectomy is performed (see Figure 34.3). Antiemetics and antinausea medication can be helpful at reducing the adverse effects of chemotherapy, and supplemental feeding methods and appetite stimulants may be considered for some patients to facilitate healing and prevent weight loss during therapy. In addition, treatment of any other problems such as renal or heart disease is important.

## Case Example

Darcie, a 9-year-old, spayed female, 4.9 kg DSH had a history of multiple small mammary tumors (largest 10 mm on pathology) found by her owner in the caudal mammary glands. Preoperative CBC, urinalysis, and chemistry profile were normal. Thoracic radiographs showed no evidence of metastases. The tumors were removed by caudal mammary gland excision. Histopathology of the masses confirmed one adenocarcinoma that was mildly infiltrative into surrounding tissues, with a "moderate" mitotic rate, and it is characterized as low grade. Other tumors were benign adenomas or noninvasive adenocarcinomas. Lymphatic vessel invasion was noted in the tumor, although the regional lymph nodes were not enlarged.

## *Case Resolution*

Due to the presence of lymphatic invasion, the risk of metastasis was considered to be very high for Darcie. For that reason, the recommended course of treatment was a chemotherapeutic course consisting of doxorubicin in combination with carboplatin. Darcie's owners refused chemotherapy. Although not needed at that time, the owners were counseled to consider surgical radical bilateral mastectomy to reduce the future risk of new mammary tumor development. This was also refused, so her owners were counseled in mammary gland palpation and to be vigilant in detecting new mammary masses and having them removed while small. Twelve months later she again had mammary nodules detected and they were removed after repeating the staging and finding no evidence of metastasis. She continued to feel well, but she had an enlarged axillary lymph node noted 2 months after the second surgery; this was found to contain metastasis of the mammary carcinoma, and her owners chose palliative care only.

# Transitional Cell Carcinoma in Dogs

## Overview

Transitional cell carcinoma (TCC) is the most common cancer of the bladder in dogs. Tumors most commonly originate in the trigone (Figures 35.1 and 35.2), but they can also occur or extend through the urethra (Figure 35.3). The symptoms are similar to those of a bladder infection, such as needing to urinate frequently but only voiding a small volume, and discomfort or pain when urinating. Infection often accompanies TCC, so urine cultures must be done, and antibiotic therapy may be needed.

TCC in dogs has a rate of metastasis of >70% at diagnosis. The most common metastatic sites are the iliac and other abdominal lymph nodes, liver, and lung (Figure 35.4). However, the life-limiting aspect of TCC is usually the impact on the pet's quality of life of the symptoms caused by the primary tumor in the bladder. Dogs that receive no treatment usually live no longer than 2 months or so, because of these symptoms and the eventual blockage of urinary outflow, meaning that they become unable to pass urine. Therefore, even when metastasis is present it is important to focus on control of the tumor in the bladder.

## Staging

Dogs with TCC may need several staging tests done before treatment. Ultrasonography of the abdomen is done to measure the size of the tumor and look for metastases within the abdomen. Radiographs of the chest should be examined for metastases to the lungs and to make sure the lungs and heart appear healthy otherwise. Urine culture should be done to check for infection and may need to be repeated later during treatment if symptoms suddenly worsen. Finally, routine blood work should be done to ensure that the dog is otherwise healthy before proceeding with chemotherapy.

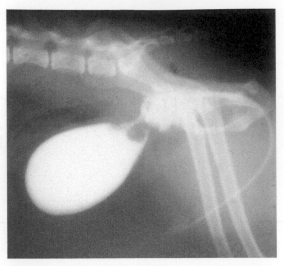

**Figure 35.1.** Contrast cystography is a fairly reliable diagnostic method for identifying a space-occupying mass in the bladder. A mass located in the trigone should raise a strong suspicion of transitional cell carcinoma. (Courtesy of Dr. Dominique G. Penninck)

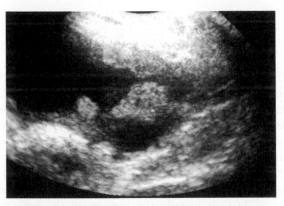

**Figure 35.2.** Ultrasonography can also be used to identify bladder masses, and it is more effective for visualizing other parts of the urinary tract and screening the rest of the abdomen for metastases. (Courtesy of Dr. Dominique G. Penninck)

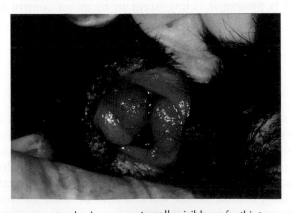

**Figure 35.3.** Urethral tumors can extend to become externally visible, as for this tumor extending into the vagina.

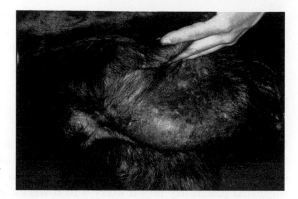

**Figure 35.4.** This dog has very enlarged inguinal lymph nodes and hindlimb edema because of metastasis from a urethral TCC.

### Dogs That Have Clinical Improvement After Treatment Live Longer

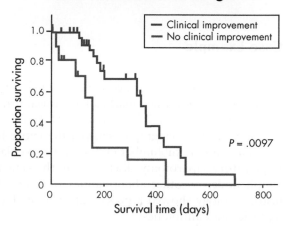

**Figure 35.5.** Kaplan-Meier survival curve showing that dogs that have any clinical improvement after treatment with chemotherapy have prolonged survival. Henry et al., *Clin Cancer Res* 9:906–911, 2003, with permission (from *Managing the Canine Cancer Patient*, Veterinary Learning Systems 2006, with permission).

## Treatment

When surgery is possible, it helps to prolong survival for dogs with TCC when followed by chemotherapy. When bulky tumor is present, the effectiveness of chemotherapy is limited. Most TCC occur in the bladder trigone (where the ureters enter the bladder), so they are not resectable.

Whether surgery is possible or not, chemotherapy has been shown to alleviate symptoms and prolong survival for many dogs with TCC. Piroxicam has the best single agent efficacy, with a reduction in tumor size of >50% in about 30% of dogs. The most common side effect of piroxicam is gastrointestinal upset, and the medication misoprostol can be given with it to reduce the likelihood of this problem. Piroxicam alone is the least expensive treatment option. The most effective chemotherapy regimen that has been reported is a combination of two medications, mitoxantrone and piroxicam. This regimen resulted in an overall 35% response rate in the measured size of the tumors in 48 dogs. Most importantly, symptomatic improvement occurred in 75% of the dogs (Figure 35.5). The average survival time in this study was 10 months, compared with 6 months with piroxicam alone. Diarrhea and kidney problems were the most common treatment complications.

Radiotherapy has been reported for this disease, but it has a high rate of serious side effects in this location (usually fibrosis), so it is not a good first-line treatment choice for dogs with bladder tumors, although it may be palliative in later stages.

## Nursing Highlights

Most dogs tolerate piroxicam well when dosed accurately and given with food. Misoprostol (at a dose of 2 to 5 μg/kg PO tid) can be used concurrently if there is vomiting or other GI signs. Piroxicam can be renal-toxic in some patients, so careful monitoring is suggested (chemistry profile every 4 to 6 weeks, at least initially).

TCC are often complicated by secondary urinary tract infections. For most patients antibiotics (based on culture results) are recommended to reduce the risk of pyelonephritis, particularly during the initial stages of chemotherapy.

## Case Example

Simba, a 7-year-old, castrated male, Scottish terrier, was presented with marked hematuria. Urinalysis confirmed marked hematuria, proteinuria, and pyuria. Serum biochemistry profile showed only mildly increased ALP. CBC showed anemia and a mild neutrophilia. Abdominal ultrasonography showed the entire bladder wall to be grossly thickened and irregular, and the sublumbar nodes were also enlarged. Thoracic radiographs were normal. Exploratory laparotomy disclosed the thickened bladder and a 5 cm × 3 cm sublumbar lymph node; no other abnormalities were noted. Biopsy of the bladder was taken and histopathology showed a poorly differentiated TCC. He was then prescribed antiinflammatories and antibiotics.

### Further Staging

Urine culture should be submitted to check for secondary infection that may be exacerbating his clinical signs.

The current ultrasonogram will serve as a baseline to determine whether there is response or progression as treatments progress. Ultrasonography should be repeated before the 3rd and 5th treatments to assess whether the treatment is helping.

### Case Resolution

Urine culture was obtained and Simba was treated with appropriate antibiotics for his secondary bladder infection. Concurrent with antibiotics, chemotherapy was started with mitoxantrone and piroxicam. Repeat ultrasonography before the third treatment found there was an approximately 75% reduction in tumor measurements, and he finished his protocol. The response was maintained at another ultrasonogram 6 months later, and he continued to be in good health.

# Pulmonary Carcinoma in Dogs

## Overview

Lung tumors are uncommon in dogs. They are seen mostly in older dogs, and the majority of dogs are more than 20 kg in body weight. Signs of the tumor include cough and problems breathing, lethargy and weight loss—although many dogs are asymptomatic.

Studies suggest that carcinogens in the environment may be a cause of lung tumors in dogs. There is higher risk for this cancer in dogs living in urban environments and a strong association between passive smoking and lung tumors in dogs. Short-nosed breeds that are exposed to second-hand smoke have an increased risk of developing primary lung tumors compared to long-nosed dogs, presumably because of the increased filtration capacity of long-nosed dogs.

## Staging

Most lung tumors are malignant, and they have often metastasized at the time they are diagnosed. The two most common sites of metastasis are other places in the lungs and the lymph nodes closest to the tumor (usually the hilar lymph nodes). Therefore, evaluation of an affected patient will include thoracic radiographs (Figure 36.1), complete blood count (CBC), biochemical profile, urinalysis, and an evaluation of regional lymph nodes by radiographs, ultrasonography, or computed tomography (CT).

The histologic *type* of tumor does not influence survival time, but the more the tumor cells resemble normal lung cells, the better the prognosis. The histologic *grade* is assessed by the pathologist. Dogs with grade 1 tumors have an average survival time of 2 years; dogs with grade 2 had an average survival of 8 months, and dogs with grade 3 tumors had an average survival of 5 days.

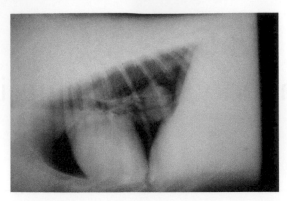

**Figure 36.1.** The initial diagnostic method for most primary lung tumors in dogs is thoracic radiography. This thoracic radiograph of a dog with a primary lung tumor shows a well-circumscribed solitary mass in the lungs.

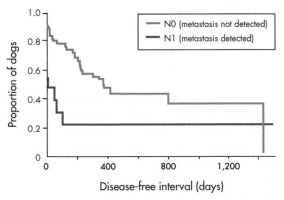

**Figure 36.2.** Kaplan-Meier survival curve showing the effect of metastasis on dogs with lung cancer. Those with evidence of spread to the lymph nodes have a much worse survival on average. McNiel et al., *JAVMA* 211:1422–1427, 1997, with permission (from *Managing the Canine Cancer Patient*. Veterinary Learning Systems 2006, with permission).

Factors influencing outcome (prognostic factors) for dogs with lung tumors include the following:

1. Dogs with tumors that have spread to lymph nodes or other sites in the lungs generally have a shorter survival expectation than dogs with no evidence of spread (approximately 12 months versus 1–2 months). The type of tumor does not influence survival times or the disease-free interval (Figure 36.2).
2. Dogs with lung tumors that are causing clinical signs at the time the tumor is detected, have a worse prognosis than if there are no clinical signs (8 months versus 18 months), even if the cancer has not yet spread.
3. Complete removal of the tumor is associated with longer survival times if the cancer is completely removed; the average survival time is 1 year, compared to 1–2 months if the excision is not complete.

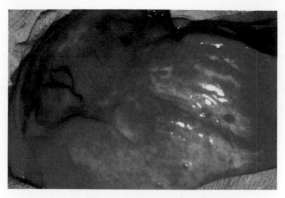

**Figure 36.3.** Surgery is the primary treatment for most dogs with lung tumors. This is a carcinoma in the right caudal lung lobe of a dog at surgery. (Courtesy of Dr. John Berg)

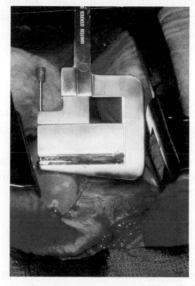

**Figure 36.4.** Automatic stapling device allows quick removal of lung lobes containing tumors. The procedure can also be done manually, but this increases surgery time. The regional lymph nodes should also be examined and biopsied during surgery, if possible. (Courtesy of Dr. John Berg)

## Treatment

As mentioned above, complete removal of the tumor as assessed by the pathologist has been shown to increase the length of survival. Therefore the surgery needs to be extensive enough to remove all cancer tissue (Figures 36.3 and 36.4). This may mean that one or more lung lobes will be removed. Radiation therapy is not really helpful in dogs with lung cancer due to risk of side effects to the normal lung tissue.

For dogs with lung tumors that have one or more poor prognostic factors listed above, systemic chemotherapy is the most likely to improve their chances of remission and survival.

## Nursing Highlights

Analgesia and soft comfortable bedding is mandatory postoperatively and should be continued at home once the patient is discharged.

Appetite stimulants, nutritional support, and antiemetic therapy may also be necessary, particularly after chemotherapy administration.

## Case Example

Jack, a 12-year-old, castrated male, 10 kg, fox terrier, was presented with a 1-month history of dyspnea and severe weight loss. Unilateral, left, pleural effusion was diagnosed on thoracic radiographs. Abdominal ultrasonography was essentially normal. Thoracic ultrasonography disclosed a left cranial lung lobe mass but no lymphadenopathy. The left cranial lung lobe was removed, allowing for complete excision of the mass. The hilar lymph nodes were not biopsied at surgery.

## *Further Staging*

A CBC, baseline chemistry panel, and urinalysis (with culture, if indicated) are always recommended for baseline staging of a pet with cancer, particularly if chemotherapy is anticipated.

It is useful to repeat 3-view thoracic radiographs as a baseline and then periodically (every 2–3 months in the absence of clinical problems) to monitor for the development of pulmonary metastases.

## *Case Resolution*

Aggressive surgery is the basis of treatment for solitary pulmonary carcinoma and had been appropriately performed. Jack's dyspnea meant that he had clinical signs of the tumor, and despite his lymph nodes being normal at the time of surgery the pathologist described the overall mitotic rate as moderate, and Jack had a grade 2 carcinoma. These factors meant that the chances of a cure for Jack with surgery alone were low and chemotherapy was considered to be the modality most likely to extend his survival.

Blood work and urinalysis was normal, and vinorelbine chemotherapy was commenced 3 weeks after thoracotomy. Jack tolerated this very well and completed his prescribed course 4 months later. At a routine recheck 6 months from surgery he was still free of recurrence.

# 37

# Chronic Lymphoid Leukemia in Dogs

## Overview

Chronic lymphocytic leukemia (CLL) is the abnormal proliferation of mature lymphocytes, which are a component of the immune system. The major diagnostic differential is acute lymphoid leukemia (ALL), where the abnormal cells are lymphoblasts. Most dogs with CLL are at least 10 years old. Most often, a pet's caregiver will notice mildly enlarged lymph nodes and the dog may have a reduced appetite and less energy. Diagnosis is based on a blood count, bone marrow evaluation, thoracic and abdominal radiographs, and other standard blood tests and urinalysis.

CLL cells live longer than normal lymphocytes. Healthy lymphocytes help fight infection. CLL cells do not. Over time, CLL cells physically crowd healthy blood cells in the blood, lymph nodes, and marrow. As the number of CLL cells grows, some dogs may have enlarged lymph nodes or an enlarged spleen, or both. This is caused by CLL cells piling up in the lymph nodes and spleen. Normally, the bone marrow produces the majority of the blood cells. CLL patients may start to feel less energy when they have fewer healthy cells and more CLL cells in the bone marrow. Tumor cells in the bone marrow can also cause the marrow to produce fewer normal cells, which aid in blood clotting and infection fighting to be available. The pet is then susceptible to bleeding and infection.

## Staging

Many otherwise healthy CLL patients are diagnosed when a routine blood test shows a higher than normal number of lymphocytes (Figure 37.1), or when an enlarged lymph node or an enlarged spleen is found during a physical exam. If there are no signs of illness, these patients are considered low risk. Further staging tests are still warranted, and thoracic radiographs and abdominal ultrasonography will help rule out the high circulating cell

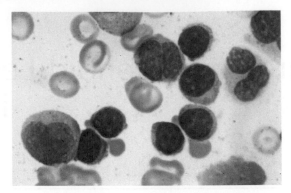

**Figure 37.1.**    Chronic lymphocytic leukemia typically presents with an increased number of circulating lymphocytes that appear well differentiated or mature; however, the counts can be very high. (Courtesy of Dr. Susan M Cotter)

count as part of lymphoma. Bone marrow aspiration cytology will help predict secondary problems due to low normal cell numbers. As always, a serum chemistry profile and urinalysis will that ensure the dog is otherwise healthy and that it does not have an underlying infection.

## Treatment

A dog with low-risk CLL will need repeat visits to the veterinarian who will check for any health changes and monitor the lymphocyte count. It is hard to tell ahead of time when a patient will need treatment. Some oncologists call this "watch and wait." Watching and waiting is hard for many caregivers to get used to. However, for low-risk CLL patients it is best not to start treatment as long as the patient feels well. The results of examinations and laboratory tests over time will help the veterinarian provide advice about when to start treatment.

The presence of a high lymphocyte count, anemia, thrombocytopenia, or clinical signs in a patient means that we would recommend chemotherapy. Chlorambucil and prednisolone are the most active agents in dogs, resulting in a median survival of 12 months (range 1 month–3 years). Some dogs will take up to 3 months to achieve a remission, *and this is common*, although symptomatic improvement usually occurs quickly.

## Nursing Highlights

There is no cure for CLL. The following are treatment goals:

1. Slow the accumulation of CLL cells.
2. Keep patients feeling well enough to carry on their day-to-day activities.
3. Protect patients from infection.

Dogs with thrombocytopenia are at risk of bleeding, and exercise should be restricted until counts are over 30,000/µl. Platelet numbers should rise with immunosuppressive prednisolone, and as the CLL responds. Even if not neutropenic, most dogs with CLL will require antibiotic therapy for potential infections due to the immunosuppression from their CLL and the immunosuppressive therapy needed to treat the CLL. Secondary infection is a common cause of morbidity and mortality in these dogs. Broad-spectrum antibiotics such as enrofloxacin should be used.

## Case Example

Baxter, an 8-year-old, castrated male, 28 kg, golden retriever was presented for wellness screening and no history of illness. A CBC showed 12,000 atypical lymphocytes, and serum globulin was normal. Repeated CBCs on four occasions over the next 5 months showed a lymphocyte count between 7,000 and 14,000 but with no other cell lines affected. The chemistry profile showed no evidence of organ damage. A bone marrow aspirate at that time showed a mild lymphocytosis but was otherwise normal. A trial course of doxycycline did not alter the CBC findings. Flow cytometry showed a homogeneous population of CD-8 T-lymphocytes, which was interpreted as lymphoid leukemia and was presumed to be CLL because the lymphocytes were consistently reported as mature. The pathologist did not mention any immature cells (with nucleoli), which would be of concern as the primary differential diagnosis would be acute lymphoblastic leukemia (ALL), a much more aggressive disease with a markedly worse prognosis. Baxter remained in otherwise good health.

## *Case Resolution*

In his situation (because his lymphocyte count was relatively stable), monthly CBCs were recommended. Over the next 5 months the lymphocyte count rose (20,000+ after 4 months and 30,000+ after 5 months); the rest of the hemogram remained normal, although the hematocrit decreased within the normal range. Although unlikely that Baxter's prognosis would have changed a lot since moving from 20,000 to 30,000 lymphocytes, it was felt that it was time to start treating him because the counts were increasing more rapidly and his hematocrit was lower. Therefore, chemotherapy with prednisone and chlorambucil was commenced. Baxter's lymphocyte count returned to normal over an 8-week period after starting chemotherapy (as is typical of this cancer). Nine months later he was still in remission, with a normal blood count.

# Section 8

## Appendices

Appendices

# Appendix 1

## BSA Conversion Charts

**Appendix 1a.** Body surface area (meter squared [m²]) conversion chart for **DOGS**

1. Make sure you have the dog's weight in *kilograms*.
2. Look up weight in kilograms on weight to body surface area (BSA) chart below.
3. Determine the dose of drug by multiplying the dosage (e.g., 30 mg/m²) by the patient's BSA (m²). **Check that this is not a dosage in mg/kg!**
4. Before preparing the chemotherapy, check the concentration (mg/ml or mg/capsule).
5. Before administering the drug, double-check the dose and results of a CBC.

| Body Weight in kg | Body Surface Area in m² | Body Weight in kg | Body Surface Area in m² |
|---|---|---|---|
| 2 | 0.16 | 8.5 | 0.42 |
| 3 | 0.21 | 9 | 0.44 |
| 4 | 0.25 | 9.5 | 0.45 |
| 5 | 0.30 | 10 | 0.47 |
| 5.5 | 0.31 | 11 | 0.50 |
| 6 | 0.33 | 12 | 0.53 |
| 6.5 | 0.35 | 13 | 0.56 |
| 7 | 0.37 | 14 | 0.59 |
| 7.5 | 0.39 | 15 | 0.61 |
| 8 | 0.40 | 16 | 0.64 |

**Appendix 1a.** *Continued*

| Body Weight in kg | Body Surface Area in m² | Body Weight in kg | Body Surface Area in m² |
| --- | --- | --- | --- |
| 17 | 0.67 | 39 | 1.16 |
| 18 | 0.69 | 40 | 1.18 |
| 19 | 0.72 | 41 | 1.20 |
| 20 | 0.74 | 42 | 1.22 |
| 21 | 0.77 | 43 | 1.24 |
| 22 | 0.79 | 44 | 1.26 |
| 23 | 0.82 | 45 | 1.28 |
| 24 | 0.84 | 46 | 1.30 |
| 25 | 0.86 | 47 | 1.32 |
| 26 | 0.89 | 48 | 1.33 |
| 27 | 0.91 | 49 | 1.35 |
| 28 | 0.93 | 50 | 1.37 |
| 29 | 0.95 | 51 | 1.39 |
| 30 | 0.98 | 52 | 1.41 |
| 31 | 1.00 | 53 | 1.43 |
| 32 | 1.02 | 54 | 1.44 |
| 33 | 1.04 | 55 | 1.46 |
| 34 | 1.06 | 56 | 1.48 |
| 35 | 1.08 | 57 | 1.50 |
| 36 | 1.10 | 58 | 1.51 |
| 37 | 1.12 | 59 | 1.53 |
| 38 | 1.14 | 60 | 1.55 |

**Appendix 1b.** Body surface area (meter squared [m²]) conversion chart for *CATS*

1. Make sure you have the cat's weight in *kilograms.*
2. Look up weight in kilograms on weight to body surface area (BSA) chart below.
3. Determine the dose of drug by multiplying the dosage (e.g., 25 mg/m²) by the patient's BSA (m²). **Check that this is not a dosage in mg/kg!**
4. Before preparing the chemotherapy, check the concentration (mg/ml or mg/capsule).
5. Before administering the drug, double-check the dose and results of a CBC.

**Appendix 1b.** *Continued*

| Body Weight in kg | Body Surface Area in m² | Body Weight in kg | Body Surface Area in m² |
| --- | --- | --- | --- |
| 0.5 | 0.063 | 5.5 | 0.312 |
| 1.0 | 0.100 | 6.0 | 0.330 |
| 1.5 | 0.131 | 6.5 | 0.348 |
| 2.0 | 0.159 | 7.0 | 0.366 |
| 2.5 | 0.184 | 7.5 | 0.383 |
| 3.0 | 0.208 | 8.0 | 0.400 |
| 3.5 | 0.231 | 8.5 | 0.417 |
| 4.0 | 0.252 | 9.0 | 0.433 |
| 4.5 | 0.273 | 9.5 | 0.449 |
| 5.0 | 0.292 | 10 | 0.464 |

# Appendix 2

## Analgesics

**Appendix 2.** Commonly used analgesics in dogs and cats

| Analgesic | Dog Dose Route and Interval | Cat Dose Route and Interval |
| --- | --- | --- |
| **NSAIDs** | | |
| Carprofen | 4.4 mg/kg PO sid OR 2.2 mg/kg PO bid OR 4.4 mg/kg SC | Postoperative: 1–4 mg/kg SC |
| Deracoxib | Postoperative: 3–4 mg/kg PO sid × 7 d Chronic: 1–2 mg/kg PO | |
| Ketoprofen | 2 mg/kg IV, SC, IM or PO initially once; then 1 mg/kg | Postoperative: 2 mg/kg SC |
| Meloxicam | 0.2 mg/kg PO, SC or IV; then 0.1 mg/kg sid | Postoperative: 0.1–0.2 mg/kg PO or SC then 0.05 mg/kg sid × 4 d Chronic: 0.1 mg/kg PO or SC; then 0.05 mg/kg sid × 4 d; then reduce to lowest effective dose |
| Piroxicam | 0.3 mg/kg PO every 24 h | 0.3 mg/kg PO every 24–48 h |

**Appendix 2.** *Continued*

| Analgesic | Dog Dose Route and Interval | Cat Dose Route and Interval |
|---|---|---|
| **Tramadol** | Up to 2–4 mg/kg PO every 6 h | 1–2 mg/kg IV |
| **Opioids** | | |
| Buprenorphine | 0.005–0.02 mg/kg IM, IV or SC every 6–12 h | Oral mucosal, IV or IM: 0.01–0.02 mg/kg every 8–12 h |
| Butorphanol | 0.2–0.4 mg/kg SC, IM or IV; OR up to 0.4 mg/kg up to every 8 h | Perioperative: 0.1–0.4 mg/kg; *not best choice* |
| Codeine | Up to 1–2 mg/kg PO every 6 h | 0.5–2 mg/kg PO titrated to effect every 6–12 h |
| Fentanyl | 3–5 µg/hr/kg patch placed every 3 d | 25 µg/h patch <5 kg half patch; >5 kg full patch; placed every 3 d |
| Morphine | 0.5–2 mg/kg IM or SC every 3–4 h | **Methadone**: 0.1 mg/kg IV; 0.3 mg/kg SC every 4 h |

# Appendix 3

## Antiemetics, Gastroprotectants, and Appetite Stimulants

**Appendix 3.**  Commonly used antiemetics, gastroprotectants, and appetite stimulants in dogs and cats

| Antiemetic | Dog Dose Route and Interval | Cat Dose Route and Interval |
|---|---|---|
| Butorphanol | 0.4 mg/kg IV 20 min prior to chemotherapy infusion<br>OR 0.4 mg/kg PO every 8 h | |
| Dolasetron (Anzemet) | 0.3–1.0 mg/kg IV, slowly. For prophylaxis: 20 min prior to and 4 h after chemotherapy infusion<br>OR 0.3–1.0 mg/kg PO every 24 h | 0.3–0.6 mg/kg IV, slowly |
| Maropitant (Cerenia) | 1 mg/kg IV, SC or PO every 24 h | 1 mg/kg IV, SC or PO every 24 h |
| Metoclopramide | 0.2–0.4 mg/kg every 6 h PO, SC or IM<br>OR 1–2 mg/kg/d as a continuous IV infusion | 0.2–0.4 mg/kg every 6 h PO, SC or IM<br>OR 1–2 mg/kg/d as a continuous IV infusion |
| Ondansetron (Zofran) | 0.1–1.0 mg/kg IV, slowly. For prophylaxis: 20 min prior to and 4 h after chemotherapy infusion<br>OR 0.1–1.0 mg/kg PO every 12 h | 0.1–0.2 mg/kg IV, slowly, 20 min prior to and 4 h after chemotherapy infusion<br>OR 0.2–0.3 mg/kg PO every 12 h (1 mg total dose) |

**Appendix 3.** *Continued*

| Gastroprotectant | Dog Dose Route and Interval | Cat Dose Route and Interval |
|---|---|---|
| Famotidine | 0.5 mg/kg PO, SC, IM, IV every 12–24 h | 0.5 mg/kg PO, SC, IM, IV every 12–24 hrs (care with IV use) |
| Omeprazole | 0.5–1 mg/kg PO every 24 h | 0.5–1 mg/kg PO every 24 hrs |
| Ranitidine | 0.5–2 mg/kg PO, IV or IM every 8–12 h | 2.5 mg/kg IV every 12 h OR 3.5 mg/kg PO every 12 h |
| Sucralfate | For large dogs: 1 gram PO every 8 hrs; for smaller dogs: 0.5 gram PO every 8 h | 0.25 gram PO every 8–12 h |

| Appetite Stimulant | Dog Dose Route and Interval | Cat Dose Route and Interval |
|---|---|---|
| Cyproheptadine (Periactin) | 0.3–2 mg/kg PO every 12 h | 0.35–1 mg/kg PO every 12–24 h |
| Diazepam | | 0.05–0.4 mg/kg IV once; then 1 mg PO once daily |
| Megestrol acetate | 0.5–1.0 mg/kg PO sid × 3–5 d; then every 2–3 d | 0.5–1.0 mg/kg PO sid × 3–5 d; then every 2–3 d |
| Mirtazapine | 0.5–1 mg/kg PO every 24 h | 0.5 mg/kg PO every 48 h |

# Appendix 4

## Antibiotics

**Appendix 4.** Commonly used antibiotics in dogs and cats

| Antibiotic | Dog Dose Route and Interval | Cat Dose Route and Interval |
|---|---|---|
| **Orally Administered** | | |
| Amoxicillin-clavulanic acid | 12.5 to 13.75 mg/kg PO every 12 h | 62.5 mg/cat (total dose) PO every 12 h |
| Cephalexin | 30–50 mg/kg PO every 12 h | 30–50 mg/kg PO every 12 h |
| Enrofloxacin | 5–20 mg/kg PO every 24 h | 5 mg/kg PO every 24 h |
| Metronidazole | 10–20 mg/kg PO every 8–12 h | 25 mg/kg PO every 12 h for 8 d |
| Orbifloxacin | 2.5 mg/kg–7.5 mg/kg PO every 24 h | 2.5 mg/kg–7.5 mg/kg PO every 24 h |
| Trimethoprim-sulphadiazine | 30 mg/kg PO every 12 h | 30 mg/kg PO every 12 h (can cause nausea) |
| **Parenterally Administered** | | |
| Cefoxitin | 30 mg/kg SC every 8 hrs OR 30 mg/kg IV every 4–6 hrs | 30 mg/kg IM or IV every 4–6 hrs |
| Enrofloxacin | 5–20 mg/kg IV every 24 h | 2.5–5 mg/kg IM every 24 h |
| Gentamicin | 6 mg/kg IV every 24 h (do not use if dehydrated) | 6 mg/kg IV every 24 h (do not use if dehydrated) |
| Imipenem with cilastatin sodium | 2–7.5 mg/kg IV or IM every 8 h for 3–5 d | 2–7.5 mg/kg IV or IM every 8 h for 3–5 d |
| Metronidazole | 15 mg/kg IV every 12 h | 15 mg/kg IV every 12 h |
| Ticarcillin-clavulanic acid | 40–50 mg/kg IV every 6–8 h | 40–50 mg/kg IV every 6–8 h |

For oral prophylaxis of patients on myelosuppressive chemotherapy, we prefer trimethoprim-sulphadiazine or enrofloxacin (orbifloxacin in cats may cause less nausea).

For neutropenic septic pets while waiting for culture and sensitivity results: broadspectrum combination therapy, such as combinations of gentamicin plus cefoxitin OR ticarcillin OR imipenem with cilastatin sodium can be used.

# Appendix 5

## Glossary of Cancer Terms

**A**

**Acute:** Symptoms occurring recently or in a short period of time

**Adenocarcinoma:** A malignant cancer arising from glandular tissue

**Adenoma:** A benign glandular tumor

**Alopecia:** Hair loss, often just whiskers in cats, most common in dog breeds that have true hair rather than fur (e.g., poodles, terriers, etc.)

**Anorexia:** Complete loss of appetite, not eating

**Antiemetic:** A drug that prevents or controls nausea and vomiting

**B**

**Benign tumor:** A cancer that does not spread from one part of the body to another and does not invade surrounding tissues

**Biopsy:** Surgical removal of a piece of tissue for examination under a microscope

**Bone marrow:** The organ found inside the bones, which generates blood cells

**Bone marrow aspiration:** Inserting a needle into a bone to sample the marrow for cytology

**Bone marrow suppression:** (see *myelosuppression*)

**C**

**Cancer:** Usually refers to a malignant neoplasm or tumor

**Carcinoma:** Cancer that starts in the skin or the organs (e.g., renal carcinoma)

**Chemotherapy:** The treatment of cancer with medications

   **Adjuvant (or adjunctive):** As a follow-up to other therapy such as surgery

   **Combination:** more than one chemotherapy agent given together at the same time or during a structured protocol

   **Neoadjuvant:** prior to other therapy in an effort to reduce the size or spread of a cancer

**Chronic:** Symptoms occurring over a long period time

**CT/CAT (computed tomography) scan:** Use of computers and x-rays to create detailed images of various parts of the body

**Cure:** Total eradication of all cancer cells

**Cystitis:** Inflammation of the urinary bladder

## D

**Drug resistance:** Method by which cancer cells develop the ability to avoid being killed by cancer chemotherapy

**Dysplasia/dysplastic:** Abnormal cell growth that is precancerous

## E

**Effusion:** Collection of fluid in a body cavity, usually between two adjoining tissues; for example, the collection of fluid between two layers of the pleura is pleural effusion

**Excision:** Surgical removal of a tumor or growth

**Extravasation:** Inadvertent leakage of injectable medication into tissue surrounding the vessel; extravasation of some chemotherapy drugs can cause significant tissue damage

## F

**Feline immunodeficiency virus (FIV):** Viral disease of cats transmitted primarily by bites between cats, which can suppress the immune system

**Feline leukemia virus (FeLV):** Viral disease of cats that can lead to the development of lymphoma

**Fine-needle aspiration (FNA):** Inserting a needle into a lesion or tissue to collect a sample for cytologic examination

## G

**Grade:** A numerical score from histologic examination that indicates how aggressive or malignant the tumor appears (high-grade is usually worse)

## H

**Hematocrit (HCT):** The percentage of red blood cells in the blood; a low hematocrit indicates anemia (similar to PCV)

**Hematuria:** Blood in the urine

**Hyperviscosity:** Sludging of blood caused by too much protein; often associated with multiple myeloma, a plasma cell cancer

## I

**Immunosuppression:** Weakening of the immune system, thereby decreasing the body's ability to fight infections and disease

**Infection:** Bacterial, viral, or fungal invasion of a body part, causing damage

**Inflammation:** Swelling, redness, warmth, and pain due to damage to tissues by cancer or treatment (not the same as infection)

**Infusion:** Delivery of fluids or medications into the bloodstream over a specified time

**Injection:** Introduction of medication into the body with a syringe and needle

    **Intracavitary:** into a body cavity e.g., abdomen or thorax

    **Intramuscular:** into a muscle

    **Intravenous:** into a vein

    **Subcutaneous:** under the skin

**L**

**Lesion:** An abnormal area, such as a lump or sore, caused by injury or disease, including cancer

**Leukopenia:** A low number of white blood cells

**Lumpectomy:** Removal of a mass without a large amount of surrounding normal tissue

**Lymph node:** Localized tissue that is part of the immune defense system; lymph nodes act as the body's first line of defense against infections and cancer

**Lymphatic system:** A network that includes lymph nodes and lymph vessels

**Lymphoblast:** an immature lymphocyte, often seen in lymphoma

**Lymphocytes:** A specific type of white blood cell; two principal types of lymphocytes (T and B) act in the immune system

**Lymphocytosis:** A high number of normal lymphocytes in the blood

**M**

**Malignant tumor:** A tumor composed of cancer cells that can spread to other parts of the body (metastasize) or invade surrounding tissues

**Mastectomy:** Surgical removal of the mammary gland (breast)

    **Simple mastectomy:** Removal of the entire breast

    **Radical mastectomy:** Removal of the entire breast along with underlying muscle and lymph nodes

**Mean:** The average number

**Median:** The middle number, often used to describe the time point at which half the patients are alive or in remission

**Metastasis:** A distant site of cancer

**Monoclonal gammopathy:** A single blood protein (globulin) produced by cancerous bone marrow cells (as in multiple myeloma)

**MRI (magnetic resonance imaging):** An advanced imaging test using magnetic energy to provide high detail images of organs and cancer in the body

**Mucosa:** The lining of the inner surface of the mouth, genitalia, and intestinal tract (also called *mucous membranes*)

**Myelodysplasia:** Disordered cell growth in the bone marrow that is preneoplastic

**Myelosuppression:** A decrease in the production or number of blood cells, often caused by either cancer or chemotherapy; severe myelosuppression may lead to infection due to low neutrophil numbers or bruising and bleeding due to low platelet numbers, very rarely anemia due to low red blood cell numbers

**N**

**Neoplasm / neoplasia:** A new growth of tissue or cells; often used instead of the word *tumor* or *cancer*

**Neutropenia:** A decreased number of neutrophils

**Neutrophil:** White blood cell that is important for fighting infections (also called *granulocyte* or *segmented neutrophil*); the **absolute neutrophil count** (not the percentage) should be assessed prior to administering myelosuppressive chemotherapy

**O**

**Oncologist:** A veterinarian or doctor who specializes in oncology

**Oncology:** The study and treatment of cancer

**P**

**Palliative treatment:** Treatment aimed at relieving pain or other symptoms of disease but not intended to cure the disease

**Pancytopenia:** Low numbers of all blood cells (red cells, white cells, and platelets)

**Pathology:** The study of disease by the examination of tissues and body fluids usually under a microscope; a specialist in pathology is a pathologist

**Petechiae:** Small blood spots in the mucosa or skin, often a sign of a low platelet count

**Placebo:** An inactive "treatment" or its effect (used in studies)

**Polyp:** A growth of tissue protruding into a body cavity that may be benign or malignant

**Preneoplastic:** Disordered growth that will become cancerous in time

**Primary tumor:** The original site of cancer

**Prognosis:** The likely outcome of a disease or the life expectancy for an individual patient

**Proteinuria:** A high amount of protein in the urine, possibly due to kidney damage

**Protocol:** Cancer treatment plan, which may involve radiation, chemotherapy, surgery, immunotherapy, and supportive care

**R**

**Radiation oncologist:** A veterinarian or doctor who specializes in the use of radiation therapy

**Radiation therapist:** A nurse or technician who treats patients with radiation therapy

**Radiation therapy (or Radiotherapy):** Treatment that damages or kills cancer cells with radiation

**Radiograph:** A diagnostic image, often called an *x-ray*

**Recurrence:** Reappearance of cancer after a period of remission

**Regression:** Reduction in size or number of cancer(s)

**Relapse:** Reappearance of cancer after a period of remission

**Remission:** Complete or partial disappearance of the signs and symptoms of cancer

  **Complete:** All detectable evidence of cancer disappears

  **Partial:** Reduction in detectable cancer by more than 50%

  **Stable disease:** Reduction of growth in cancer that is less than 50% or increase of less than 25% (may just be due to measurement errors or changes in inflammation)

**S**

**Sarcoma:** Malignant tumor of supporting tissue, such as bone, muscle, or cartilage

**Sepsis:** Overwhelming systemic infection, potentially fatal, may occur when a chemotherapy patient is severely neutropenic

**Staging:** Determination of extent of cancer in a patient's body

**Systemic disease:** A disease that affects the whole body instead of a specific organ

**T**

**Tumor:** An abnormal overgrowth of cells; tumors can be either benign or malignant, often used instead of the word *cancer*

**U**

**Ultrasonogram:** The use of high-frequency sound waves for the purpose of imaging and examining internal body structures (also *ultrasonography, ultrasound,* or *sonogram*)

## V

**Venipuncture:** Placing a needle or catheter into the vein to obtain blood samples or administer intravenous medication or fluids

**Vesicant:** An intravenous medication that, if leaked into tissues, could cause pain, swelling, and/or tissue damage

## W

**White blood cell count (WBC, WBCC):** Number of white blood cells in a blood sample; not to be confused with neutrophil count; WBCC is not sufficient to assess effects of chemotherapy, and the **absolute neutrophil count** should be assessed

# Appendix 6

# Chemotherapy Drug Information: Quick Reference

### Actinomycin-D

| | |
|---|---|
| **Available:** | 0.5 mg/ml vials |
| **Route:** | Give intravenously with over-the-needle catheter. Reconstitute vial with 1.1 ml sterile water or 0.9% NaCl (without preservative, which may cause a precipitate). Discard unused solution. Administer into the injection port of a running saline infusion over 5–10 minutes. **Vesicant when given perivascularly.** |
| **Dosage:** | According to protocol, at intervals of every 1–3 weeks. |
| **Storage:** | Room temperature. |
| **Monitor:** | Do not administer if neutrophil count is less than 3,000/µl. |

### BCNU

| | |
|---|---|
| **Available:** | 100 mg vial with 3 ml sterile alcohol diluent. Add 27 ml of sterile water for injection to diluted drug to yield a solution containing 3.3 mg BCNU per ml. |
| **Route:** | Give intravenously with over-the-needle catheter. BCNU should be infused over 20–30 minutes. |
| **Dosage:** | Every 3–4 weeks according to protocol. |
| **Storage:** | Refrigerate. |
| **Monitor:** | Do not administer if neutrophil count is less than 3,000/µl. |

### Bleomycin

| | |
|---|---|
| **Available:** | 10 ml vial (1 mg = 1 USP unit = 1,000 IU) |
| **Route:** | Subcutaneously or intralesionally |
| **Dosage:** | Every week or according to protocol |
| **Storage:** | Refrigerate. |
| **Monitor:** | Leucopenia and thrombocytopenia are very rare. |

## Carboplatin

| | |
|---|---|
| Available: | 450 mg in 45 ml, or 150 mg in 15 ml |
| Route: | 10 mg/ml diluted to a total dose volume of 25 ml (cats) or 50 ml (dogs) with 5% *dextrose* and give slow IV push over 15–20 minutes |
| | **OR** |
| | undiluted, slowly inject into the injection port in the line of a running infusion of 5% *dextrose* over 15–20 minutes |
| Dosage: | According to protocol, usually every 3 (dogs) to 4 (cats) weeks |
| Storage: | Refrigerate. |
| Monitor: | Do not administer if neutrophil count is less than 3,000/µl. |

## CCNU (Lomustine)

| | |
|---|---|
| Available: | 10 mg, 40 mg, 100 mg capsules, or as capsules reformulated to 2.5 mg or specific dosage for cats and small dogs |
| Route: | Orally |
| Dosage: | According to protocol, usually every 4 weeks (dogs) to 6 weeks (cats) |
| Storage: | Room temperature. |
| Monitor: | Do not administer if neutrophil count is less than 3,000/µl. Monitor ALT level; do not administer if elevated. |

## Chlorambucil

| | |
|---|---|
| Available: | 2 mg tablets, or reformulated from a compounding pharmacy for cats and small dogs |
| Route: | Orally |
| Dosage: | According to specific protocol |
| Storage: | Refrigerate. |
| Monitor: | Do not administer if neutrophil count is less than 3,000/µl. |

## Cisplatin

| | |
|---|---|
| Available: | 50 mg vials, reconstituted to 1 mg/ml |
| Route: | IV with catheter, or intracavitary given according to protocol |
| Dosage: | **DO NOT USE IN CATS.** |
| | **Dogs:** every 3–4 weeks, but dose varies with weight and according to specific protocol. Precede with dolasetron (Anzemet) or maropitant (Cerenia). |
| Administration: | Cisplatin *must* be preceded and followed by an established diuresis protocol. Needles or intravenous sets containing aluminum parts that may come in contact with solution should not be used for preparation or administration. Aluminum reacts with cisplatin, causing precipitate formation and loss of potency. |
| Storage: | Refrigerate. |
| Monitor: | Renal function (serum creatinine and urine specific gravity) before each treatment. Do not administer if renal insufficiency. |

## Cyclophosphamide

| | |
|---|---|
| Available: | 25 mg (U.S. only) or 50 mg tablets or 100 mg (U.S. only) and 500 mg vials. Reconstitute vials with 0.9% NaCl to concentration of 20 mg/ml. |

**Route:** PO or IV with catheter as a slow (2–5 minutes) push. Furosemide (2–4 mg/kg once) is given IV after a saline flush between the drugs or PO at the same time.

**Dosage:** See specific protocol; dose varies with route and interval and species.

**Storage:** Store unreconstituted drug at room temperature. Reconstituted drug is stable for 6 days when refrigerated.

Tablets should never be split due to inconsistent distribution of active drug throughout the tablet **and due to risk of exposure to handler.**

**Monitor:** Do not administer if neutrophil count is less than 3,000/µl.

## Dacarbazine (DTIC)

**Available:** Reconstitute 100 mg vial with 9.9 ml of sterile water. Reconstitute 200 mg vial with 19.7 ml of sterile water.

**Route:** *Give intravenously with over-the-needle catheter.* Dilute with 0.9% NaCl to a 1 : 1 ratio; given as a slow intravenous push.

**OR**

*intravenously as an infusion over 4–5 hours.* Dilute into 250–1000 ml of 0.9% NaCl.

**Dosage:** According to protocol after pretreatment (20 minutes before starting infusion) with dolasetron (Anzemet) or maropitant (Cerenia)

**Storage:** Refrigerate.

**Monitor:** Do not administer if neutrophil count is less than 3,000/µl.

## Doxorubicin

**Available:** 10 mg, 20 mg, 50 mg vials at concentration of 2 mg/ml

**Route:** Give intravenously with over-the-needle catheter. Administer into the injection port of a running saline infusion over 10–20 minutes (rate of about 1 ml per minute).

Rapid infusion may be associated with histamine release and anaphylactoid reaction (restless, urticaria, vomiting, even collapse); slow infusion avoids this.

Use plain normal saline for flushing—heparin may cause a precipitate to form.

**Vesicant when given perivascularly.**

**Dosage:** Dosage usually every 3 weeks according to protocol

**Storage:** Refrigerate and protect from light.

**Monitor:** Do not administer if neutrophil count is less than 3,000/µl.

## Gemcitabine

**Available:** 200 mg, 1 g vials for reconstitution with 0.9% NaCl to 40 mg/ml

**Route:** IV with over-the-needle catheter

Give as an intravenous infusion over minutes to hours.

**Dosage:** According to protocol. **Unlike many other drugs** *longer infusion times equate to increasing dosage levels.* It is uncertain if the dose-time relationship is linear, but most oncologists assume that it is.

**Storage:** *Store* unopened vials at room temperature. Once reconstituted, refrigerate and use within 24 hours.

**Monitor:** Do not administer if neutrophil count is less than 3,000/µl.

## Ifosfamide

| | |
|---|---|
| Available: | 1 g and 3 g vials (mesna is included in the package). Reconstitute with 0.9% NaCl to 50 mg/ml |
| Route: | IV as continuous infusion diluted in 0.9% NaCl and given over 30 minutes. Must be preceded and followed by 0.9% NaCl fluid diuresis. Additionally, to help prevent hemorrhagic cystitis, mesna should be administered in three doses, each equal to 20% of the ifosfamide dose. Mesna is given as an IV bolus at the start of pretreatment diuresis and 2 and 5 hours after ifosfamide infusion. |
| Dosage: | According to protocol, but minimum dose interval is every 2–3 weeks. |
| Storage: | Store at room temperature. Reconstituted solution is stable for 6 weeks refrigerated. |
| Monitor: | Renal function (serum creatinine and urine specific gravity) before each treatment. Do not administer if renal insufficiency. Do not administer if neutrophil count is less than 3,000/μl. |

## L-asparaginase

| | |
|---|---|
| Available: | 10,000 IU vials for reconstitution. Reconstitute with 2 ml 0.9% NaCl slowly (will form bubbles if mixed too fast) to final concentration of 5,000 units/ml. |
| Route: | Subcutaneously or intramuscularly (*Can cause an anaphylactic reaction if given intravenously; rarely by other routes.*) |
| Dosage: | According to protocol, but minimum dose interval is weekly. |
| Storage: | Refrigerate. Use within 8 hours of reconstitution and discard unused solution. Do not use unless clear. *Some sources suggest that refrigerated solution may be stable for 7–10 days.* |
| Monitor: | L-asparaginase alone is not bone marrow suppressive, but it can be very myelosuppressive when given at same time as vincristine. |

## Melphalan

| | |
|---|---|
| Available: | 2 mg tablets, or reformulated from a compounding pharmacy for cats and small dogs. **Do not split pills due to risk of exposure to handler.** |
| Route: | Orally |
| Dosage: | According to protocol |
| Storage: | Refrigerate. |
| Monitor: | Do not administer if neutrophil count is less than 3,000/μl. |

## Mitoxantrone

| | |
|---|---|
| Available: | 10 mg, 20 mg, 25 mg vials at concentration of 2 mg/ml |
| Route: | Give intravenously with over-the-needle catheter. Administer into the injection port of a running saline infusion over 5–10 minutes. Use normal saline for flushing—*no heparin*—may form a precipitate. |
| Dosage: | According to protocol, but usually every 2–3 weeks |
| Storage: | Refrigerate. |
| Monitor: | Do not administer if neutrophil count is less than 3,000/μl. |

## Procarbazine

| | |
|---|---|
| Available: | 50 mg capsules or reformulated from a compounding pharmacy for cats and small dogs |

| | |
|---|---|
| **Route:** | Orally |
| **Doseage:** | In combination with other drugs, usually daily for 14 days |
| **Storage:** | Room temperature. |
| **Monitor:** | Do not administer if neutrophil count is less than 3,000/µl. |

## Vinblastine

| | |
|---|---|
| **Available:** | 10 mg vials at concentration of 1 mg/ml |
| **Route:** | IV with catheter as a bolus injection<br>**Vesicant when given perivascularly** |
| **Dosage:** | According to protocol, but usually every 1–2 weeks |
| **Storage:** | Refrigerate. Reconstituted solution is stable for 30 days refrigerated and if protected from light. |
| **Monitor:** | Do not administer if neutrophil count is less than 3,000/µl. |

## Vincristine

| | |
|---|---|
| **Available:** | 1 mg, 2 mg, 5 mg vials at concentration of 1 mg/ml |
| **Route:** | IV with catheter as a bolus injection<br>**Vesicant when given perivascularly** |
| **Dosage:** | According to protocol, but usually every 1–2 weeks |
| **Storage:** | Refrigerate. Reconstituted solution is stable for 30 days refrigerated and if protected from light. |
| **Monitor:** | Do not administer if neutrophil count is less than 3,000/µl. Vincristine alone is not very myelosuppressive, but it can be very myelosuppressive when given at same time as L-asparaginase. |

## Vinorelbine

| | |
|---|---|
| **Available:** | 10 mg, 50 mg vials at concentration of 10 mg/ml Dose should be further diluted in 0.9% NaCl to 5 ml total volume. |
| **Route:** | IV with catheter as a slow bolus injection over 5 minutes<br>**Vesicant when given perivascularly** |
| **Dosage:** | According to protocol, but usually every 1–2 weeks |
| **Storage:** | Refrigerate. Reconstituted solution is stable for 30 days refrigerated and if protected from light. |
| **Monitor:** | Do not administer if neutrophil count is less than 3,000/µl. |

# Index

Printed and bound by CPI Group (UK) Ltd, Croydon, CR0 4YY

27/10/2024

14580243-0003